HEALING RECIPES
JENNA CARPENTER

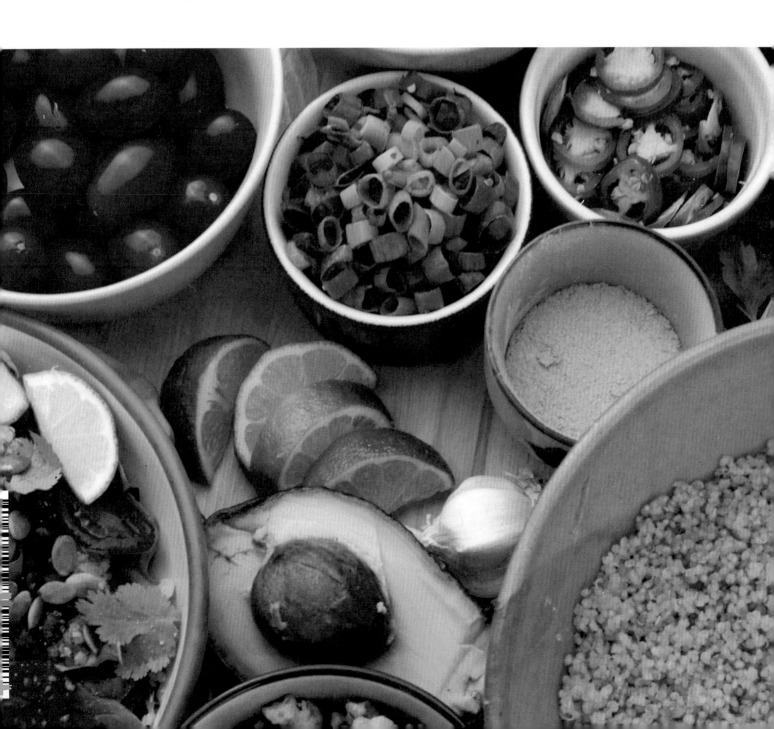

Healing Recipes

My Journey

I can remember spending hours in the kitchen when I was a kid. I loved to create, cook, and bake. Growing up in the south I ate a typical American diet, loaded with processed foods like mac-and-cheese, Cheez Whiz, tuna fish salad, canned soups and vegetables. On the weekends, I would bake cakes and cookies. During the week, I would insist on not only making my own lunch, but my mom's too. My palate developed by the age of 18, and I began truly appreciating the food I ate. When I moved to San Diego, I fell wildly in love with Mexican food. When I worked late-night shifts, burritos were routinely my jam when I got off work.

In addition to developing my palate, I also developed a deep love for yoga practice. My practice led me to Santa Cruz, where I met a teacher who guided me through the physical practice but also made a big impact on the way I perceived life. I can remember at the end of one class, she had us sit in a circle and gave each of us a single raisin. She instructed us first to observe it, and then to place it in our mouths without chewing. After some time we were allowed to chew, ever so slowly. It was a practice in mindful eating, and one of the most powerful moments in the evolution of my lifestyle and diet transformation.

A few years later, I started teaching yoga in San Diego. I loved everything about it - the practice, the community of teachers, students, and like-minded folk. As I built my teaching practice and developed other areas of my life, there was a voice inside of me that craved adventure and exploration of other cultures. I could no longer resist my desire to travel - so I packed my bags! While abroad, I noticed some alarming skin discoloration in a sensitive area of my body. I immediately went for a biopsy and was diagnosed with lichen sclerosus. To add insult to injury, I broke out in hives all over my body from the traumatic experience at the doctor's office. My body was clearly in shock and I needed to get my histamine levels back to normal.

This experience was the catalyst for regaining my health. It was then that I decided to change my diet, which felt like the only thing I had control over. Initially, I incorporated more raw foods and eventually removed all dairy, gluten, caffeine, and meat. I wanted to heal from the root of the cause and not simply place a band aid on the problem. I did endless amounts of research on lichen sclerosus and discovered it was linked with autoimmune disease. That's when I decided it was in my best interest to do a much needed cleanse.

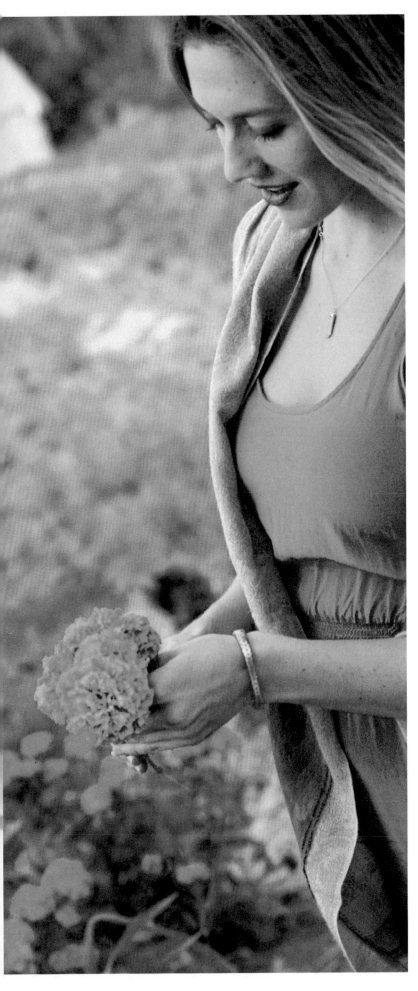

This cleanse wasn't just about food though, it was about looking at the areas of my life that were out of sync. I began meditating regularly, journaling, discovering my purpose, deepening my relationships, and viewing life from a holistic approach. This process helped me realize that my healing greatly depended on balance.

I went back to school at The Institute for Integrative Nutrition, where I learned how to balance my life and diet. While completing my studies, I was living abroad in Argentina, where I started to spend most of my free time in the kitchen. I found a new way to drop in and be present.

As a meaningful moment in my transformative journey through food, I created these recipes for you to share with family and friends. I encourage experimenting with each one, adding a twist or modification as you please. That's exactly how I came up with many of these recipes - just by playing in the kitchen! Cooking can be an amazing, creative outlet and delicious medicine for the body and soul. I hope these healing foods bring you much joy and balance! Happy cooking - be well, and get after it!

Jenna Carpenter

Before diving deep into the kitchen with this book as a handy copilot, be sure to clean, clear, and create a space that is sacred and that you enjoy being in!

Take a few hours to focus on getting rid of things. Start by clearing out any expired products. Next, read the labels on food items in the refrigerator and pantry. If there is any unfamiliar vocabulary on the label, get rid of it. Any processed or expired food you have, throw it away.

Stick to **whole**, **fresh**, **organic**, and even **local** foods. Here is a list of the basics to have in your kitchen.

Fresh Fruit & Vegetables
Berries
Bananas
Apples
Lemons
Avocados
Tomatoes
Spinach
Sweet Potatoes
Bell Peppers
Onion
Garlic

Grains
Quinoa
Millet
Buckwheat
Gluten-free Oats
GF Crackers, such as
Mary's Gone Crackers
Rice Crackers

Seeds & Nuts
Sunflower seeds
Pumpkin seeds
Chia seeds
Flax seeds
Sesame seeds
Almonds
Cashews
Almond butter
Tahini

Protein
GF tempeh
Tofu
Lentils
Garbanzo beans
Black beans

Seasonings & Herbs
Cayenne
Paprika
Cumin
Turmeric
Coriander
Oregano
Fresh Parsley & Cilantro
Cinnamon
Sea Salt & Pepper
Nutritional Yeast
Coconut Oil
Extra Virgin Olive Oil
Coconut Amino Acids
Raw Apple Cider Vinegar
Dijon Mustard
Organic Veggie Broth
Unsweetened Almond Milk
Stevia
Honey
Maple Syrup

Food Schedule

The following food schedule is an outline of "A day in the life" while on a whole foods cleanse. Keep in mind everybody's body is different, which means, do what works best for you. Adjust portion size accordingly. I have listed a few options below. You may eat more or less, depending on what feels right for you.

Prevent "binge eating" by eating smaller portions every few hours. This is also a great way to keep your blood sugar levels stable and your energy steady. Do your best to eat MINDFULLY and SLOWLY.

In general, stick to homemade meals and steer clear of processed foods: food in a can or box, frozen, etc. Eating this way is better for you and the environment (cutting down on waste and packaging that processed foods come in).

Also, it is good to know where your food comes from. Connect with your local farmers and farmers' markets. Or even better, grow it yourself!

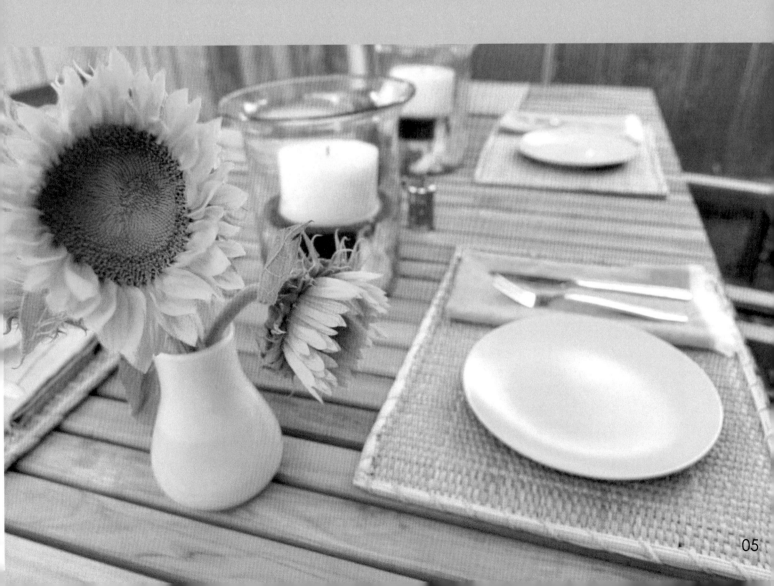

Sample Menu

Wake-Up
- drink a glass of warm H2O, with lemon
- follow up with one more glass of water/herbal tea

Breakfast
- eat within 45 min. of waking
- start with ½ of a grapefruit
- ½ cup of oatmeal or chia pudding
- green smoothie

Midmorning Snack
- ½ avocado with herbs and squeeze of lemon
- handful of raw veggies with 2 tbsp hummus
- green apple with 2 tbsp of nut butter
- 10 rice/seed crackers with 2 tbsp hummus or nut butter

Lunch
- 2 generous cups of mixed greens salad with 4-6 oz of protein (**options:** clean animal protein or try tempeh, tofu, or beans), and ¼ of an avocado
- 2 cups steamed veggies with spices and Bragg's/Coco Aminos, 4-6 oz. protein, ¼ cup of quinoa
- 2 cups of homemade soup, add 1 handful of spinach on top

Afternoon Snack
- ¼ cup quinoa, served with ½ cup steamed and seasoned veggies (kale, broccoli, cauliflower) sprinkled with sunflower or pumpkin seeds
- green smoothie or green juice
- ½ cup of kale salad (or your choice)

Dinner
Eat before 8pm or 2 hours before bed.
- 1 cup of cooked black bean pasta (or quinoa...looking for GF) served with pesto sauce and 1-2 cups chopped raw/steamed spinach. Garnish with fresh herbs.
- add some cherry tomatoes, and 1 tbsp chopped nuts
- 2 cups salad and 1 cup soup
- 1-½ cups of Mexican quinoa with 1-2 cups salad or steamed greens

Before bed, make a protein shake with protein and water/nut milk. I recommend ½ water & ½ nut milk. (If you participate in resistance training, this can help your muscles recover faster and increase your muscle mass.)

How to eat, what to eat, the way you eat, and whom you eat with is your choice. Choose what is best for you, but really think about it first! As I mentioned before, every body is different. And ultimately, the decision is yours. **Eat with purpose, pleasure, and balance.**

The following recipes are vegan and gluten-free. Originally, this book was written for participants on a whole foods cleanse, however, they can be enjoyed by everyone of all ages!

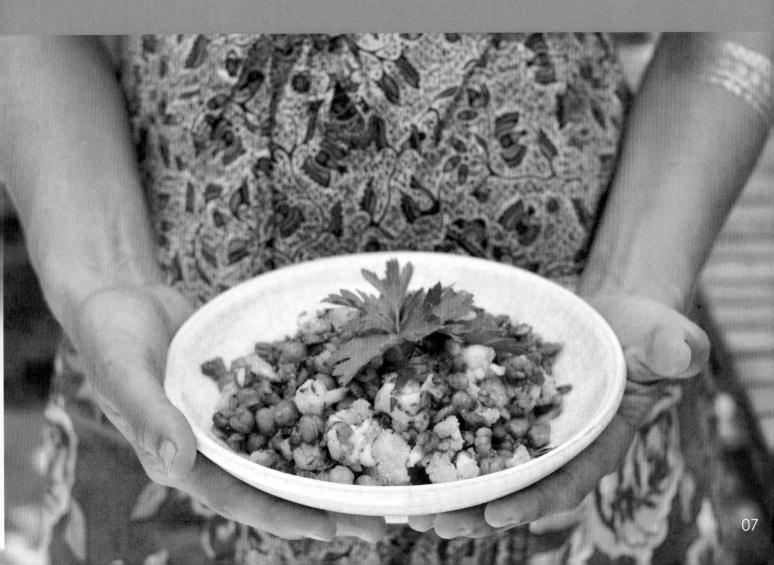

CONTENTS

Drinks

Hydration

But first, let's hydrate! Hydrate before breakfast. Start the day with one big glass of warm water with lemon (or apple cider vinegar) and 1 tsp of chia seeds. Hydration is extremely important for overall health, physical performance, glowing skin, consistent bowel movements, and is a form of flushing out toxins in the body.

Consider investing in a glass or stainless steel water bottle that you enjoy drinking from. Take time to spice up your water and get creative! It keeps hydration more exciting. Experiment with adding citrus, apples, berries, cucumbers, and herbs like mint, rosemary, basil, cardamom, or ginger. Be consistent with water intake and drink every hour, if possible. Be aware of where your water comes from, its value and how clean it is. Ideally, drink the most water in the first part of the day. And stop drinking several hours before going to bed. This will help with less bathroom trips in the middle of the night and increase a more restful sleep.

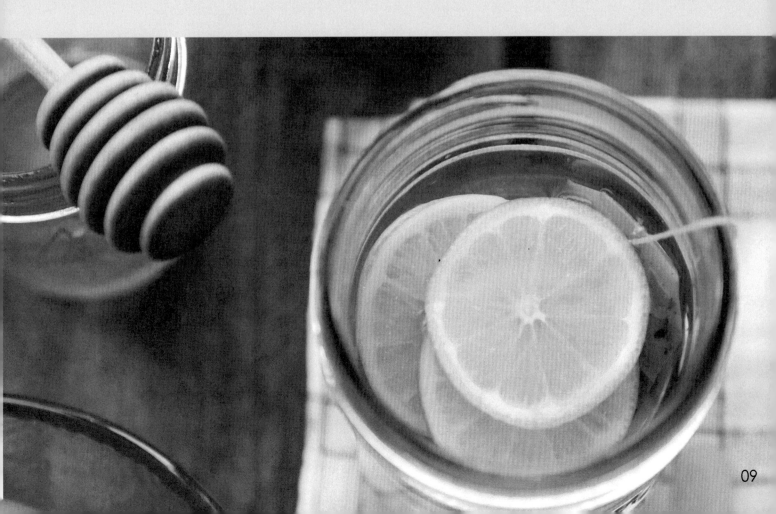

Homemade Almond Milk or Coconut Milk

Pour hot water over coconut/nuts, let stand for 15 minutes, or until cool. Place ingredients in blender, power on high for 30 seconds-1minute and strain in big bowl, using a cheesecloth. Use left-over fiber for baking (raw protein balls, smoothies, chia pudding, or oatmeal).
Optional: *add cinnamon or vanilla. Use the coconut milk for oatmeal or to add to herbal teas during detox. Some of the following recipes call for it. Almond milk is best enjoyed when fresh, otherwise it separates when stored in the fridge (don't worry, it's still good!) Just throw back in the blender before using.*

- 1 cup shredded coconut or soak raw nuts (overnight or minimum 4 hours)
- 3 cups boiling water
- liquid vanilla stevia to taste *optional

Extra Easy Coconut Milk

Blend on low, the following ingredients together. Other **options** *are to add a few drops of liquid stevia, a dash of vanilla, and/or cinnamon. Good for 3-4 days.*

- 1 can of organic coconut milk
- 3-4 cups of water

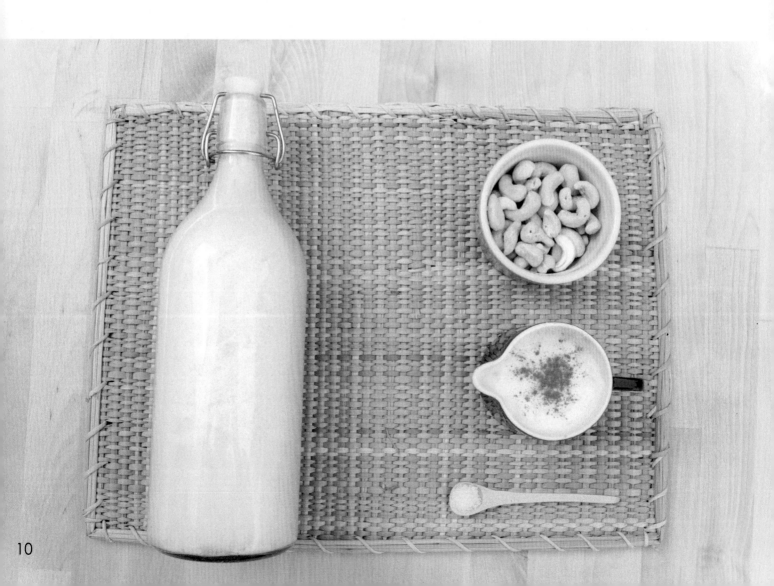

Agua Con Gas

Place the following ingredients in a mason jar, stir, and enjoy.

- 24 oz of sparkling water
- squeeze of lemon/lime
- 2-5 drops of liquid vanilla stevia

Agua Con Chia

Place the following ingredients in a mason jar. Pour in chia seeds, one tablespoon at a time, to prevent clumping. Shake jar with lid when seeds settle to the bottom.

- 24 oz of water
- 5 tbsp of chia seeds
- 4-5 strawberries
- 4 drops of liquid vanilla stevia
- ½ squeeze of lemon/lime/orange juice

Strawberry Lemon Tonic

Put the following ingredients in a mason jar and mash with wooden spoon, add water. Let sit a few hours or overnight.

- 24 oz of water
- 10 strawberries cut in half without stems
- 1 sliced lemon

ACV Health Cocktail

Combine the following ingredients in a sealed container and shake. Pour over ice, and enjoy anti-inflammatory, immune boosting, detox, and weight-loss benefits.

- 8-16 oz. water
- 1 tsp lemon juice
- 1 tsp raw apple cider vinegar
- ¼ tsp powdered ginger
- ¼ tsp powdered turmeric
- ½ tsp cinnamon

Green Lemonade Juice

After juicing the following ingredients, add water or coconut water into 24 oz mason jar, shake, and serve. Drink within an hour to receive maximum benefits and freshness.

- 1 bunch of kale stems
- 2 lemons
- ¼ inch of fresh ginger root
- 1 apple

Going Green

After washing, trimming and chopping the following ingredients, place them in a blender. Add water if needed. **Optional:** *add lemon juice, pinch of sea salt or lemon stevia to taste.*

- 3 cups coconut water
- 2 cups water
- 1 granny smith apple, cut into quarters then cored, but not peeled
- 4 stalks celery, with leaves
- 3 large romaine lettuce leaves
- ½ large avocado
- ¼ cup chopped cilantro or parsley

Classic Breakfast Smoothie

Combine the following ingredients in blender and enjoy.

1 cup almond milk or coconut milk
1 cup frozen blueberries, raspberries or acai berries
1 banana
1 tbsp coconut oil
1 scoop protein powder
1 tbsp hemp seeds
1 tsp maca powder
1 tsp Vitamineral green powder or handful of spinach

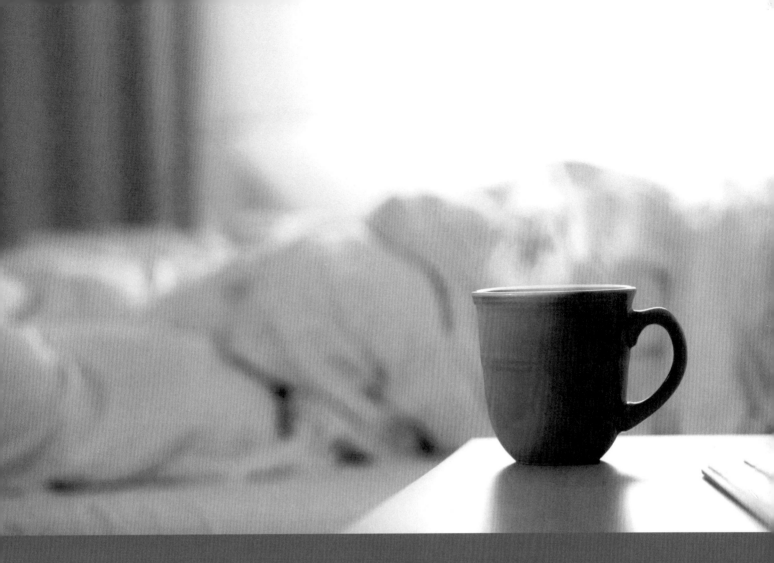

Turmeric Ginger Tea

Bring 1-2 cups of water to a boil. Add ginger and turmeric, and let simmer for 5-10 minutes. Strain water into a tea cup and add honey to sweeten. Enjoy hot or cold.

- ¼ tsp ginger root, grated
- ¼ tsp turmeric root, grated
- 1 tsp honey (optional sweetener)

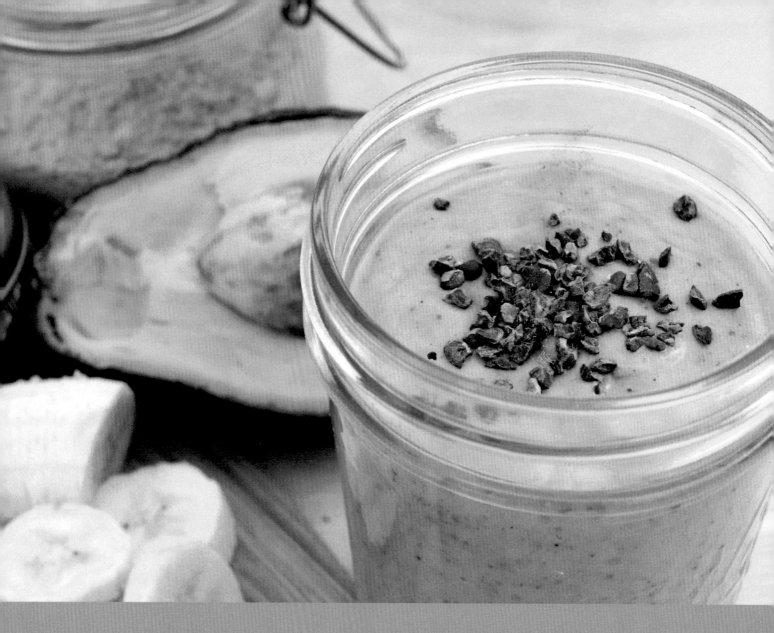

Avocado Smoothie

Combine the following ingredients in blender and enjoy.

- ½ cup almond milk
- ¾ cup filtered water
- ½ avocado
- 1 banana
- 1 scoop vanilla protein powder
- 1 tbsp coconut oil
- 1 tsp Vita Mineral Greens
- ½ tsp maca powder
- 1 tbsp cacao nibs
- 1 pitted date or stevia
- 1 pinch of pink salt

Almond Dream Machine

Combine the following ingredients in blender and enjoy. Serve in a chilled glass to make it extra fancy. This is a great post workout!

- 1 cup almond milk
- ½ cup water
- 1 tbsp almond butter
- ½ tsp vanilla
- 1 tsp Vita Mineral Greens
- ¼ tsp cinnamon
- 1 scoop protein powder *optional
- a few ice cubes *optional

Cherry Delight

Combine the following ingredients in blender and enjoy. Add a splash of water or ice, if desired. Serve in a chilled glass to make it extra fancy.

- 1 cup coconut water
- 1 cup spinach
- ½ cup water
- ¼ cup cherries
- 2 tbsp raw cashews
- 1 scoop protein powder

Bethany's Famous Smoothie

Combine the following ingredients in blender and enjoy.

- 2 cups almond milk
- 1 cup frozen blueberries
- ½ cup ice
- 1 banana
- 3 leaves of kale
- 1 tbsp peanut butter

Breakfast

Breakfast is a big deal. So why not incorporate healthy, healing foods? It's the first opportunity of the day to fuel the body. After sleeping, it is important to break the fast! By eating something in the morning, it helps to stabilize blood sugar levels. This means you will have more energy, and your brain will turn on sooner rather than later.

Keep in mind, it is important to choose foods best for you always, to create sustainable and vibrant health. Everybody's body is different, so eat accordingly, and take time to experiment with diet and lifestyle. These two components influence one another.

If eating breakfast is challenging and new for you, eat something light even if you aren't hungry, for at least one week. It takes time to develop, so if you aren't hungry initially, stick with it. Keep breakfast light, and know that eating something is better than nothing.

In our culture today, we are busy. However this isn't an excuse for eating on the go. I am as guilty as anyone else when it comes to eating on the way to my next activity. Break the habit and make breakfast a priority. Place devices in another room. Sit down and be present with your food by taking time to really look at what you are putting into your body, smell it, taste the different flavors, and enjoy by savoring every bite. Our digestion starts the moment we start chewing, so let eating be a ritualistic practice.

Breakfast Ritual

Take a good look at your food.
Bless your food and give gratitude for every bite.
Pay attention to how you eat, what you are eating, where it came from.
Enjoy food with good company.
And always, eat slowly.

On a side note, pay attention to food combination. It is recommended to eat fruit separate from other foods, to maintain optimal digestion. Foods have different digestion rates, and fruit tends to digest quicker. When fruit is consumed with grains, it can cause the fruit to ferment and this can cause gas or bloating. When you eat fruit, eat it before any grains so it can digest and pass out of the stomach before it ferments.

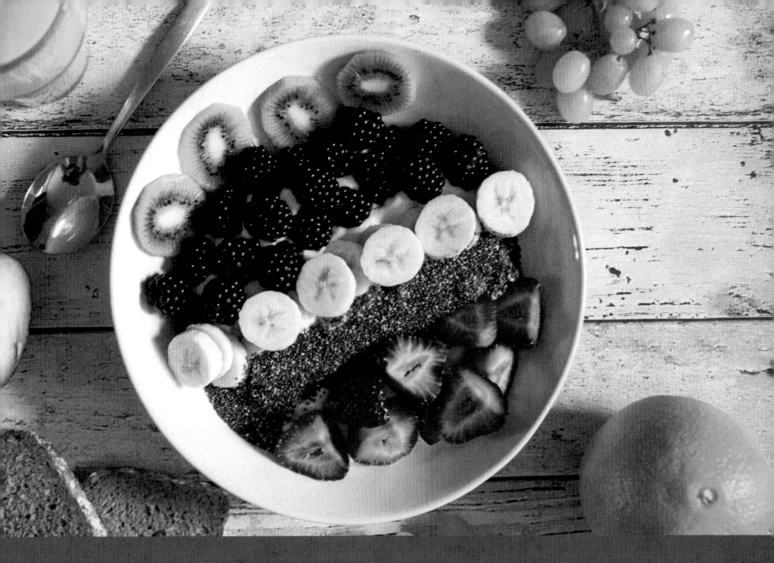

Cha Cha Cha Chia Puddin'

- 2 cups homemade coconut milk
- ½ cup chia seeds
- 1 tsp vanilla extract
- 1 tsp vanilla liquid stevia
- ½ tsp cinnamon
- pinch of pink salt

Stir all the ingredients together, until combined. Taste and adjust sweetener to your preference. Let sit 5 minutes in fridge. Stir and pour into 2-3 serving glasses. Refrigerate 30 minutes until set.

Optional: *add a tbsp of nut butter, nuts, or berries.*

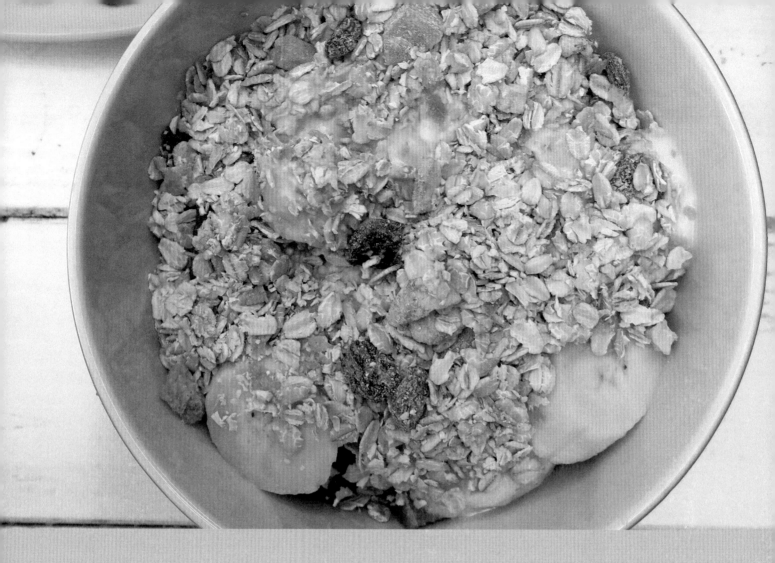

Good ole' Oatmeal

- ½ cup gluten free oats
- 1 tbsp pumpkin seeds
- 1 tbsp almond butter
- 1 tbsp molasses
- ½ tsp pink salt
- ½ tsp coconut oil
- ½ tsp cinnamon
- water or coconut milk
- stevia or honey to taste

*Soak oats overnight in filtered water or coconut milk. In the morning, heat 1/4 cup water in small saucepan on medium heat. Place soaked oats and add the rest of the ingredients. Add sweetener, like a few dates, stevia, maple syrup, or ½ tsp molasses. Tip: While soaking oats overnight, cover with towel and place in fridge. **Optional:** add chia seeds or ground flax seeds for extra omegas and fiber. This meal can be enjoyed hot or cold!*

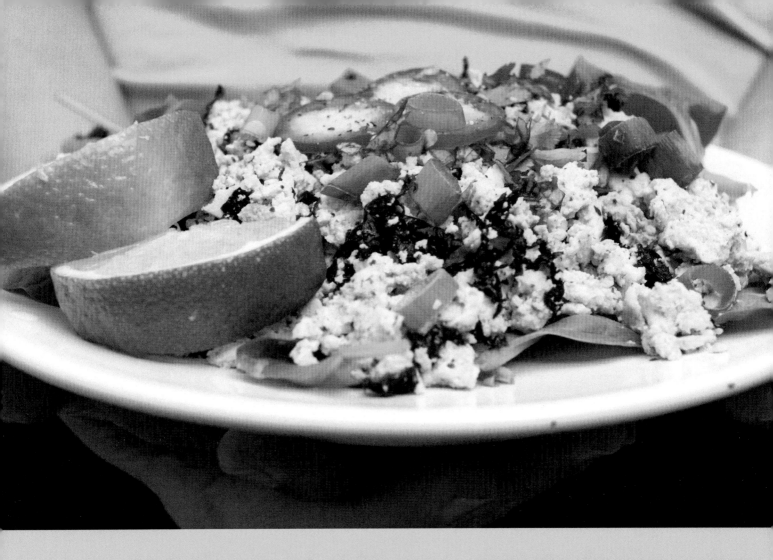

Nori Ginger Tofu Scramble

- 3 sheets nori
- 1 package tofu
- 2 tbsp nutritional yeast
- 1 tbsp coconut oil
- 1 tsp minced ginger
- 1 tsp turmeric
- 1 tsp tamari

Cut nori sheets into very thin one inch strips (scissors work best). Heat coconut oil in a skillet. Crumble tofu and add to skillet, once oil is heated. Simmer until tofu is heated. Stir in nori, ginger, nutritional yeast and tamari. Cook for 5 more minutes or until fully heated through. Sprinkle on toasted sesame seeds for added flavor, and garnish with fresh cilantro. This scramble is great for breakfast, lunch, or dinner!
***Tip:** For even more flavorful tofu, soak it overnight in spices.*

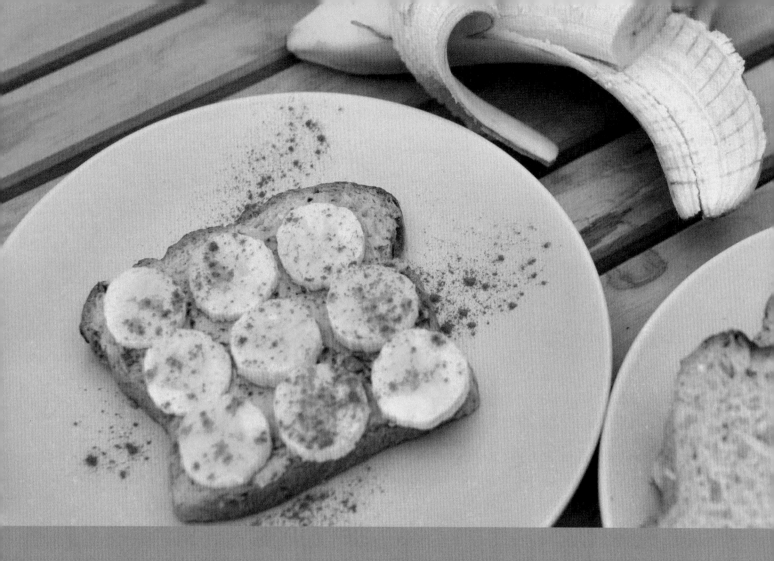

Almond and Honey Toast

- 1 piece of gluten free bread
- 1-2 tbsp almond butter, or peanut butter

Toast bread, and spread favorite nut butter on it, drizzle with raw honey and cinnamon. Add thinly sliced apples, bananas, or strawberries for extra flavor.

Avocado and Tomato Toast

1 piece of gluten free bread
1 sliced avocado
1 sliced tomato

Toast bread and spread sliced avocado on it. Add sea salt, black pepper, cayenne, fresh cilantro and lime juice. Drizzle a teaspoon of extra virgin olive oil for extra flavor.

Options: add sprouts, sliced tomato, basil, etc.

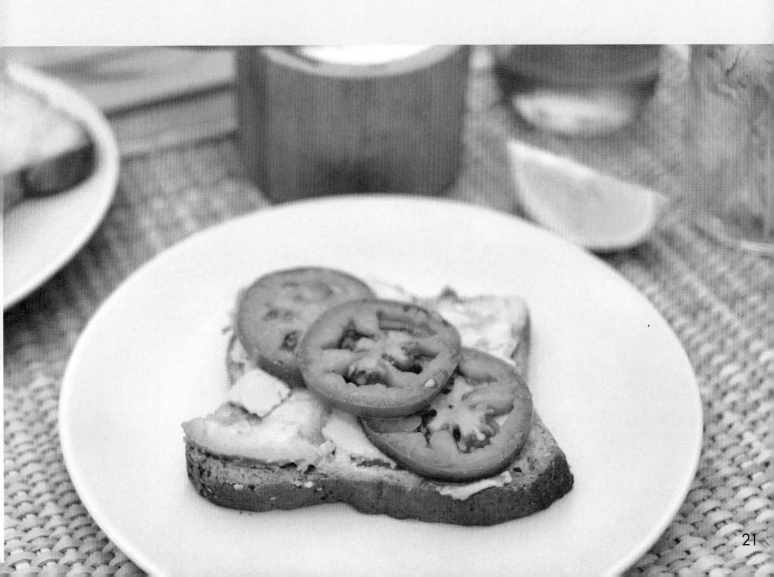

Veggie Pie

Part 1 - Crust

- 2 cup almond meal
- ½ cup arrowroot flour
- ½ tsp baking soda
- ½ tsp sea salt
- 6 tbs extra-virgin olive oil
- 1 flax egg (2 tbsp ground flax, 4-5 tbsp filtered water)
- 1 tbsp filtered water
- 2 tsp grated lemon zest
- 1 tbs juice

Heat oven to 350.
After mixing ingredients together, place in pie dish. Distribute the dough evenly (start from the middle and press out to edges) with spatula or fingers. Place in oven for 10 minutes.

Part 2 - Filling

- 2 ½ cups of raw, cashews (soak overnight or a few hours)
- ¼ cup filtered water
- 6 tbsp nutritional yeast
- 4 tbsp extra-virgin olive oil
- 2 tbsp lemon juice
- 1 tbsp minced garlic
- 1 tsp sea salt

Blend ingredients in food processor or high-powered blender, until creamy.
Optional: *add spices like cayenne, paprika, turmeric, or even ½ a red pepper. Place cheese in pie crust.*

Part 3 - Topping

- 1 medium zucchini
- 2 medium Roma tomatoes
- 2 tbsp lemon juice
- 2 tbsp extra-virgin olive oil
- 1 tsp sea salt
- ½ tsp cayenne
- ½ tsp oregano

Slice zucchini and tomatoes in medium bowl, and stir in other ingredients. Then, place zucchini and tomatoes on top of CASHEW CHEESE. Place your veggie pie in the oven for 20-25 minutes on 350. Take it out and add freshly chopped herbs like parsley, cilantro, or green onions.

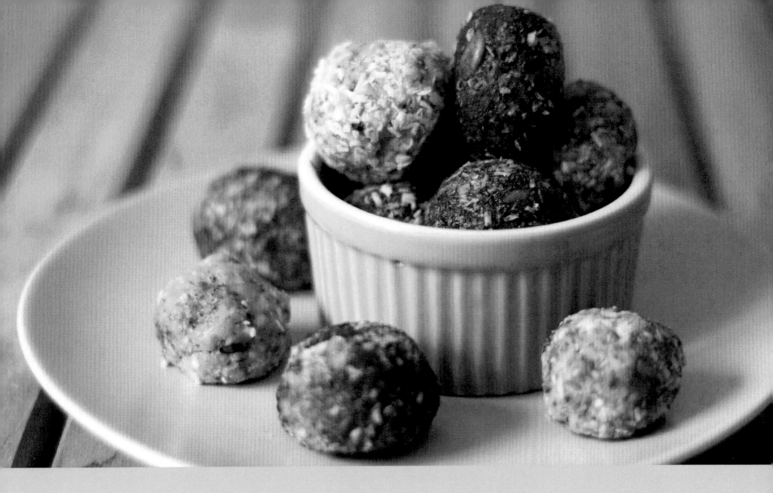

Protein Balls

- ¾ cup peanut butter
- ½ cup shredded coconut
- ¾ cup almond flour
- ¼ cup ground pumpkin seeds
- 1 tbsp ground flax seed (mix with 4 tbsp water/almond milk)
- 1 tsp melted coconut oil
- 1-3 tbsp maple syrup
- ¼ tsp pink salt
- liquid stevia to taste

Optional Toppings

- 1 tbsp chia seeds
- 1-2 tbsp hemp seeds
- 2 tbsp shredded coconut

Mix all ingredients in medium size bowl (except toppings).
***Option:** add protein powder, cacao powder, nibs, and chopped nuts. Roll into small balls and then cover with toppings. For easy clean up, place balls on wax paper (either on cookie sheet or large plate).*

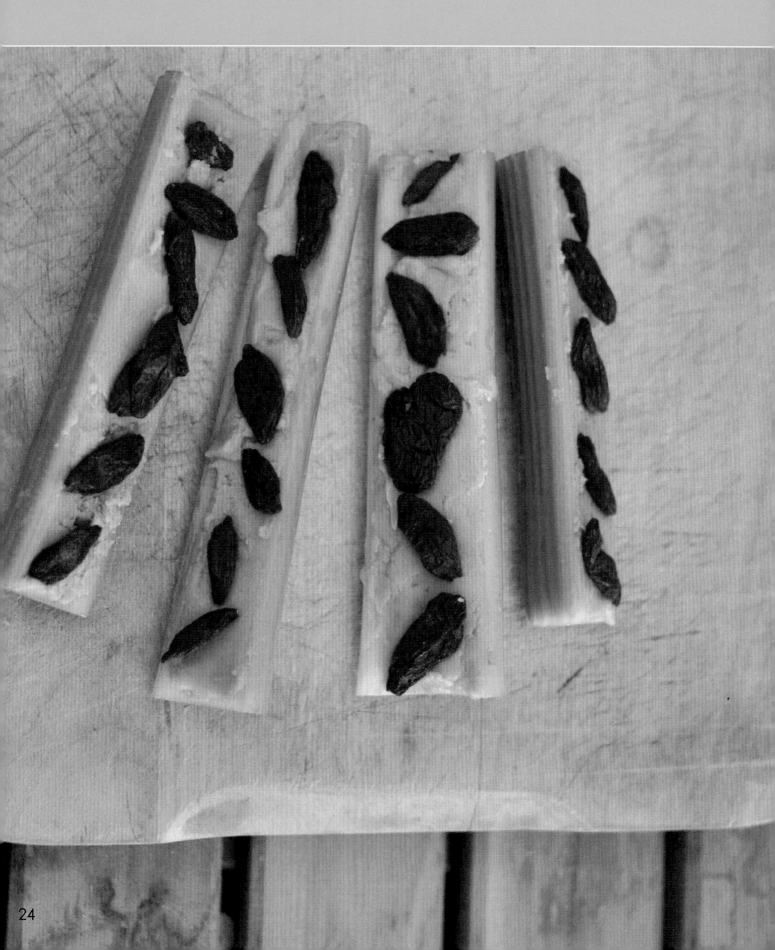

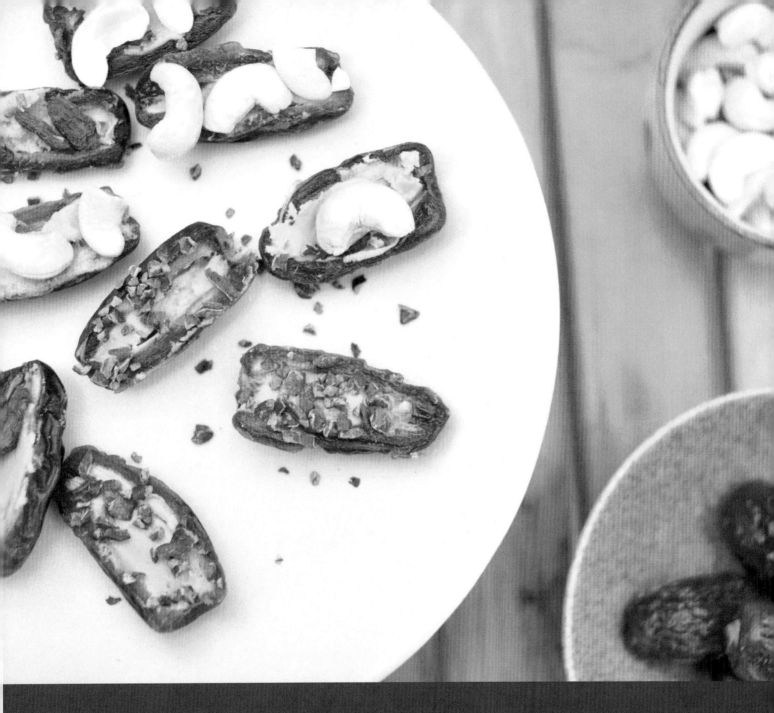

Dates & Nut Butter

Cut dates in half and add favorite nut butter. Sprinkle with cashews, cacao nibs, goji berries, etc.

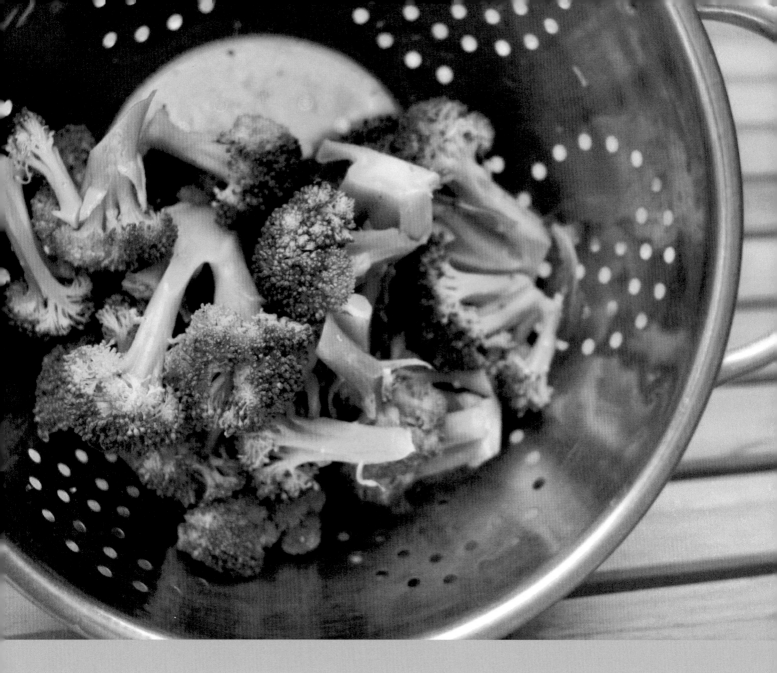

Steamed Broccoli

- 6 cups chopped broccoli
- ½ cup vegetable broth
- 1 tsp of coconut oil
- 2 tbsp minced garlic
- 2 tbsp minced ginger
- 1 tbsp tamari sauce
- 1 tbsp apple cider vinegar

Heat saucepan on medium with coconut oil. Add garlic, ginger, broth, tamari, and vinegar. Let boil, then put broccoli in and cover. Steam for 5-8 minutes.
Option: *sprinkle with nutritional yeast.*

Roasted Carrots & Sweet Potatoes with Cilantro, Lime, and Avocado Topping

Part 1. *Roast Carrots & Sweet Potatoes. Heat oven to 400. Place potatoes and carrots in large mixing bowl, drizzle oil and stir seasonings in. On large cookie sheet, place wax paper down and add veggies, leave about ½ inch between each piece and roast for 40 minutes.*

- 8 medium sized carrots, cut in 2 inch pieces
- 1 large sweet potato, roughly chopped (or sliced into wedges)
- 1 tsp cumin
- 1 tsp cayenne
- 1 tsp black pepper
- 2 tsp pink salt
- 1-2 tbsp extra virgin olive oil or avocado oil

Part 2. *Heat 1tsp of coconut oil in small pan. Once melted, add chopped walnuts (soaked for 2 hours and drained) and pepitas for 1-2 minutes. The pepitas start to brown quickly.*

- 1 tsp coconut oil
- ¼ cup raw walnuts
- ¼ cup raw pepitas

Part 3: *In small bowl, stir the following ingredients together.* **Option:** *to add finely chopped (raw) jalapeño. Combined all three parts into large bowl. Serves 4-6, save ½ cup portions to eat as snack, to place over chopped spinach and cherry tomato salad, or over microgreens or sprouts.*

- 1 avocado, chopped
- 1-2 tbsp lemon juice
- ¼ cup chopped cilantro
- pink salt to taste

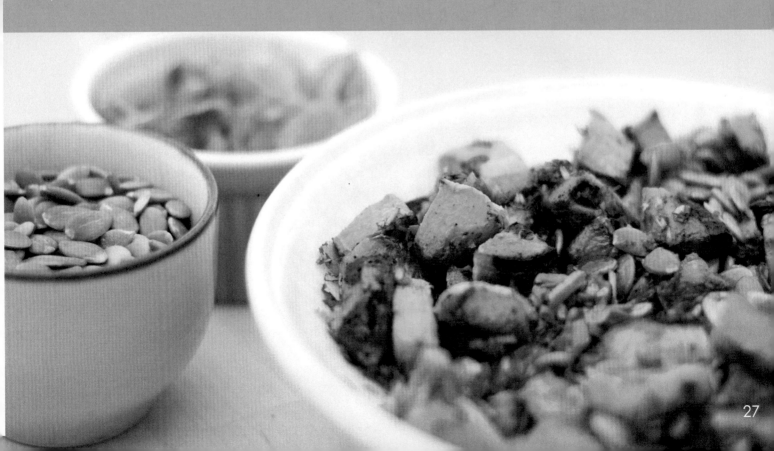

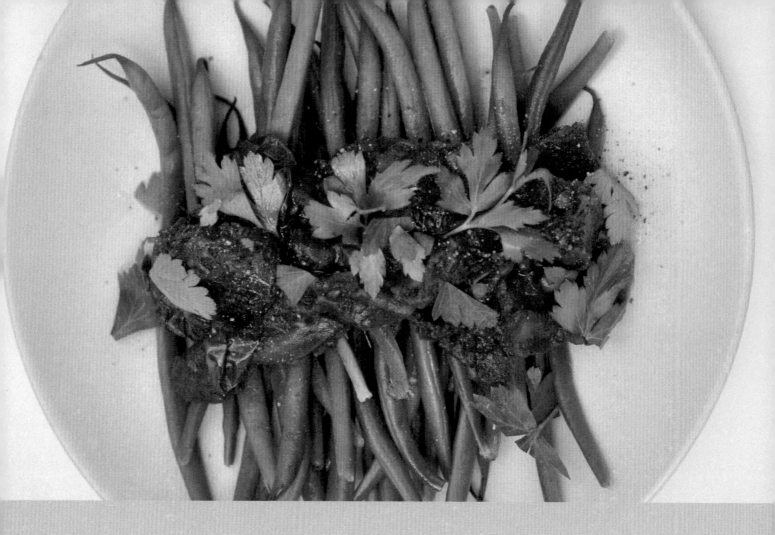

Green Beans in Tomato Sauce with Fresh Parsley

- 1 medium onion, chopped
- 1 pound green beans, trimmed and chopped in half
- 1 can of roasted tomatoes or 1 package of cherry tomatoes, freshly roasted
- ¼ cup of water or vegetable broth
- 1 bay leaf
- 2 tbsp minced garlic
- 1 tsp pepper
- 1 tsp cayenne
- 2 tsp avocado or coconut oil
- ½ cup of freshly chopped parsley
- pink salt, extra virgin olive oil, and lemon juice to taste

In a medium saucepan, saute onions on medium-low heat in 1 tsp of avocado oil (or coconut oil), with a pinch of salt. After about 5 minutes, add garlic. Once the onions are translucent, add green beans, the rest of seasonings, roasted tomatoes, and water/ vegetable broth. Let simmer for 45 minutes, with lid on. Remove from heat, and let cool for 15 minutes. Drizzle EVOO, fresh lemon juice, salt to taste, and place parsley on top.

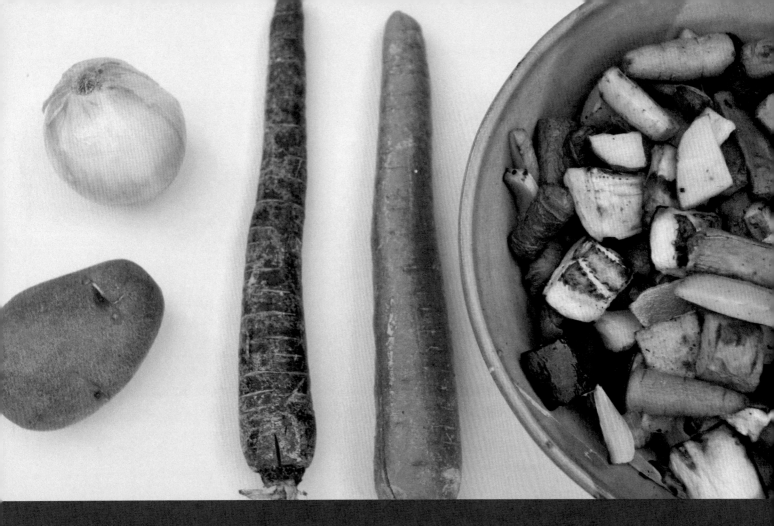

Roasted Veggies Recipe

- 2 cups asparagus
- 2 cups eggplant
- 2 cups butternut squash
- 2 cups sweet potatoes
- 1 cup red onion
- 1 cup red pepper
- 4 tbsp extra virgin olive oil or coconut oil (melted)
- 2 tbsp minced garlic
- 1 tsp sea salt
- 1 tsp pepper
- other seasonings of choice

Preheat oven to 450. Peel and roughly chop vegetables, then place in large bowl. Drizzle oil and add seasonings, toss to coat. Arrange on two baking sheets with wax paper. Spread the vegetables out and roast for 30 minutes. Check on them after 20 minutes and move them around with wooden spoon. Add 10 minutes if needed.

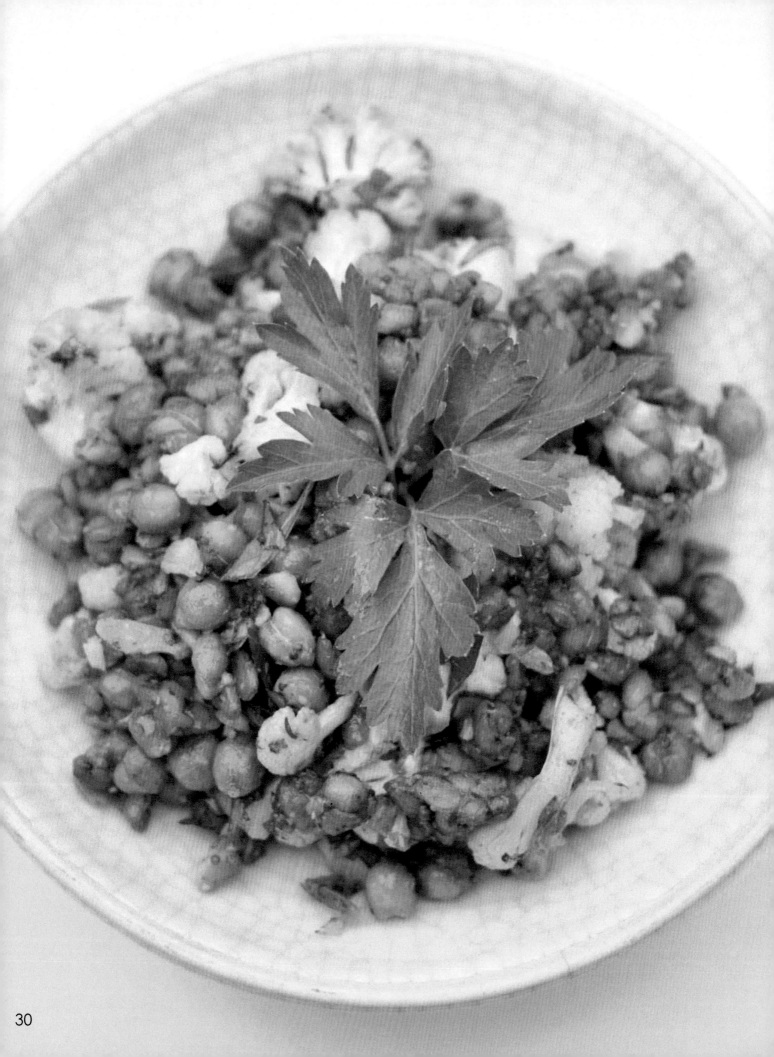

Roasted Chickpeas, Cauliflower, & Tempeh

- 1 head of cauliflower
- 1 can rinsed chickpeas (any beans will work)
- 1 package tempeh
- ¼ cup extra virgin olive oil
- 1 tbsp seeded mustard
- 1 tbsp dijon mustard
- 1 tbsp unfiltered apple cider vinegar
- 1 tbsp lemon juice
- ¼ tsp cayenne, paprika, and cumin (¼ tsp of each)
- pinch of salt/ground pepper
- ¼ cup chopped parsley/cilantro

Part 1. *Preheat oven to 400. Chop cauliflower into bite-size pieces. Stir in medium bowl with chickpeas and crumbled tempeh. Add 2 tbsp extra virgin olive oil, salt, cayenne, paprika, and cumin. Place cauliflower and chickpeas/ beans in a large pan with wax paper and place in oven for 35 minutes.*
Tip: *I like to add the tempe h after the first 10 minutes that the cauliflower and beans have been in the oven.*

Part 2. *Mix mustard, vinegar, ¼ cup of extra virgin olive oil, salt and pepper to- gether in large bowl. Add a bit of honey, if you would like to add a little sweet to your salty. After you take out the cauliflower, chickpeas, and tempeh, place in large bowl (with other ingredients) and toss. Add the parsley, while it's still warm.*

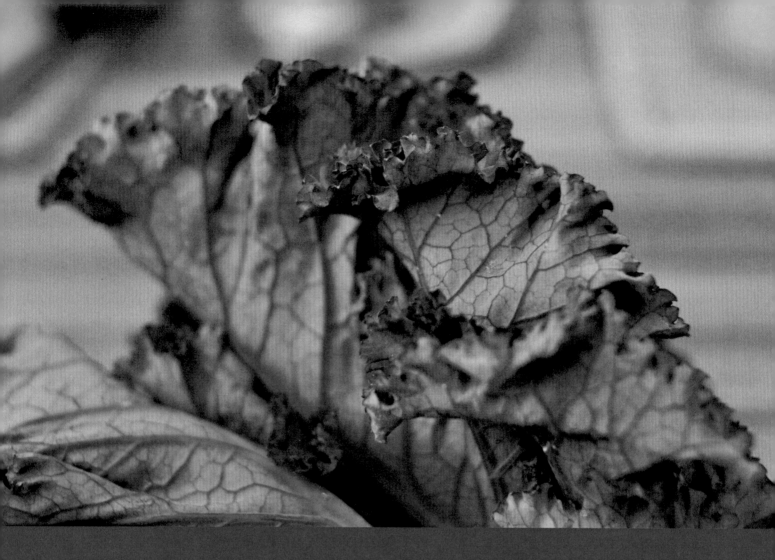

Kale Chips

- 1 bunch kale
- 3 tbsp extra virgin olive oil
- 2 tsp salt and pepper
- 2 tbsp nutritional yeast

De-stem and chop or tear kale into large 2" pieces. Massage in grape seed oil and lay flat onto cookie sheet with wax paper. Sprinkle salt, pepper and nutritional yeast. Bake at 350 for about 10-12 minutes or until crispy.

Entrées

Quinoa/Grain Tip

Quinoa is an awesome, superfood that can be made at the beginning of the week so you can add it to salads, veggie dishes, or anything else. To give it more flavor, I cook my quinoa in veggie broth with a ton of spices (ginger, cayenne, cumin, turmeric, etc). Here is a delicious recipe option...

First, place 1 tbsp of coconut oil in pot to melt, add ¼ cup onions and 3 cloves of garlic, finely chopped. When the onions look and taste soft (become more translucent), put 2 cups of veggie broth in pot on medium high heat. Once it is boiling, add 1 cup of quinoa and reduce heat. Cook time is about 15-20 minutes. Add in your favorite spices like ginger, cayenne, cumin, and turmeric. Once it's done, turn off and let cool.

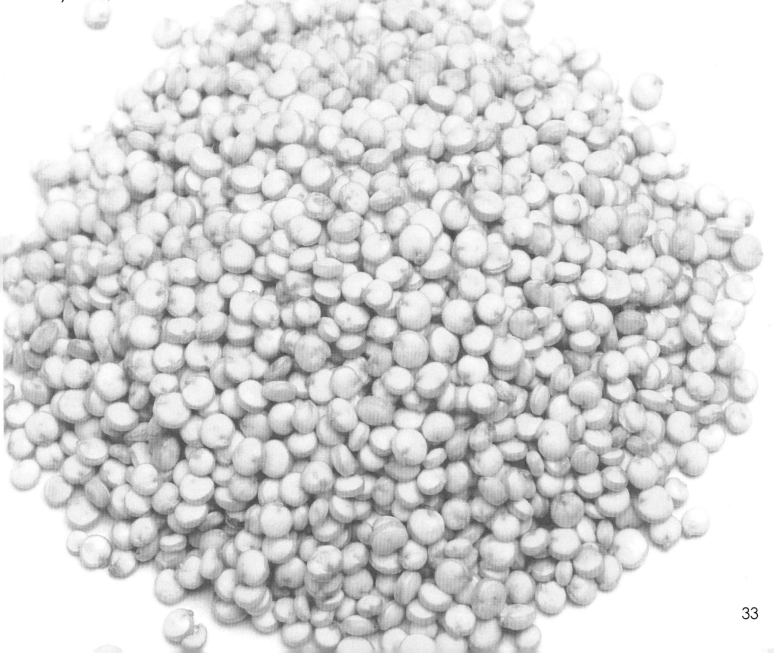

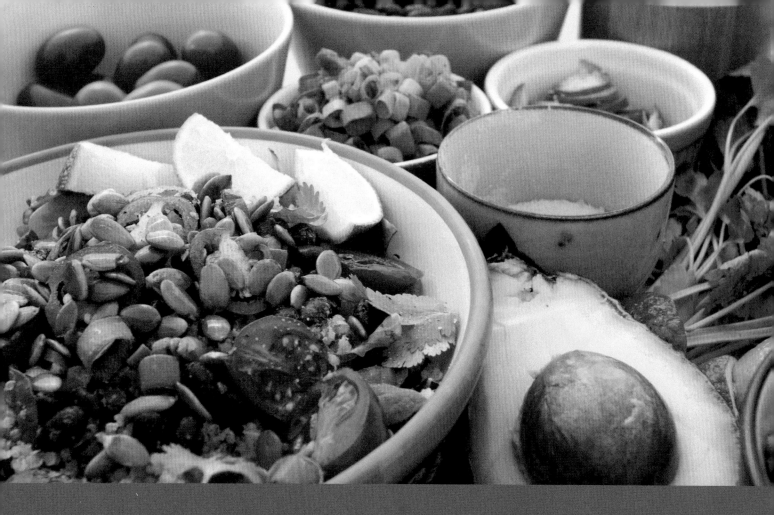

Mexican Quinoa

- 2 cups cooked quinoa
- 1 can rinsed black beans
- 1 package of cherry tomatoes
- ¼ cup chopped parsley
- ¼ cup chopped cilantro
- ¼ cup chopped green onions
- juice of 1 lemon
- 1 chopped green pepper
- 1 chopped red pepper
- 2 tbsp Braggs or coconut aminos
- 2 cups steamed kale or raw spinach
- 3 tbsp sunflower seeds
- 3 tbsp pumpkin seeds

Place ingredients in a big bowl and mix. For extra flavor, add cumin, paprika, cayenne pepper, salt & pepper. Add 3 tablespoons nutritional yeast for some creamy texture, chopped avocado for garnish, raw jalapeno (finely chopped), and seeds. This dish can be eaten cold or warm on top of greens or with sauteed vegetables.

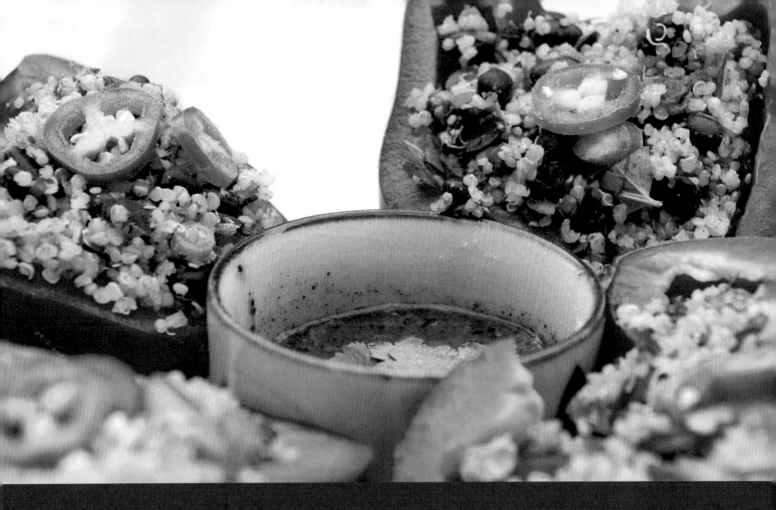

Quinoa Stuffed Peppers

- 4 large red peppers
- 2 cups cooked quinoa
- 1 cup rinsed black beans
- 1 tbsp nutritional yeast
- ½ cup Homemade Salsa
- 2 tsp chili powder/mix of your favorite spices
- 2 tbsp melted coconut oil

Heat oven to 375, lightly grease baking dish with coconut oil. Mix above ingredients (not the topping options) in a bowl. Cut peppers in half and remove seeds. Lightly brush peppers with melted coconut oil. Mix quinoa, black beans, yeast, salsa and seasonings in medium bowl. Then, scoop ingredients into halved peppers, place in baking dish and cover with foil. Increase oven temperature to 400, place peppers in oven and bake for 15-20 minutes. Let cool and add toppings of choice. To reheat, place peppers in the oven on 350 for 15 minutes.

Recommended Topping Options:
sliced avocado, fresh lime, cilantro, green onion, salsa

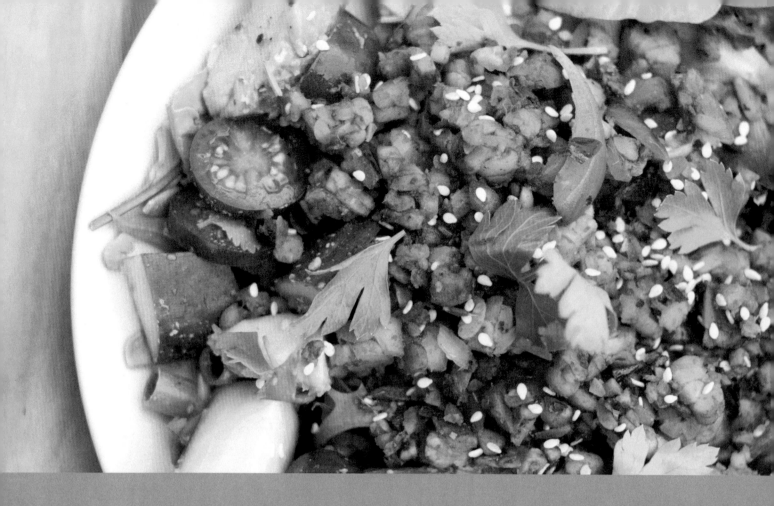

Tempeh Tacos

- 1 package (8 ounces) organic tempeh, crumbled
- 2 cups chopped greens
- 2 tsp coconut oil
- 3 tbsp tomato paste
- 2 tbsp sesame seeds
- 2 tbsp apple cider vinegar
- 1 tbsp tamari
- 1 tbsp fresh chopped jalapeño
- 2 tbsp fresh chopped red onion
- 2 tsp maple syrup
- ½ tsp cayenne
- ½ tsp cumin
- avocado slices

Heat 2 tsp of the oil in a large skillet over medium heat. Add the crumbled tempeh and sauté until lightly brown, stirring frequently. Meanwhile in a small bowl, whisk together the remaining oil, Worcestershire sauce, tomato paste, sesame seeds, vinegar, and syrup. Pour the sauce over the tempeh and let the mixture cook for about 3 to 4 minutes or until the sauce is absorbed into the tempeh. To assemble the tacos, place a spoonful of meat on a lettuce leaf and top with the avocado slices.
Option: add Homemade Salsa (see recipe in Sauces).

Black Bean and Quinoa Burgers

- ½ cup cooked organic red quinoa
- 1 can organic black beans, drained
- 2-4 tbsp water
- 2 tbsp extra-virgin olive oil
- 1 tbsp nutritional yeast
- 1 tbsp ground flax seed
- ½ tsp cumin
- ½ tsp ground black pepper
- ½ tsp paprika
- ½ tsp sea salt

Preheat oven to 400 degrees. In small bowl, mix water and ground flax seeds. Let sit for a few minutes. In a medium-sized bowl, combine 1 tbsp of olive oil with remaining ingredients. Use a fork or your hands to mash the beans and mix thoroughly until the mixture is a paste-like texture, adding flax/water combo (it's a great binding ingredient). Divide the mixture into 4 equal balls, and form each into a burger-sized patty. In a medium-sized oven-safe pan, cook patties over high heat in ½ tbsp coconut oil for one minute on each side, until lightly browned. Place pan into the oven and bake for 15 minutes. Serve as desired.

Crunchy Kelp Noodles

- 4 ounces kelp noodles (glass noodles)
- ⅛ cup fresh herbs of your choice (mint, basil)
- 4 tbsp shredded carrots
- 1 cucumber, sliced into thin rounds
- 4 tbsp rice vinegar/ ACV
- 3 tbsp tamari
- 2 tbsp sesame seeds
- 1 tbsp maple syrup

Mix together kelp noodles and carrots. In a separate bowl, whisk together vinegar, maple syrup, and tamari. Add cucumber and mix well. Garnish with herbs and sesame seeds and serve. Note: Kelp noodles can be found in the health food store.

Pasta Salad

Served warm or cold. Add "Ashley's Special Sauce" for extra flavor.

- 1 package of cooked (penne) Brown Rice Pasta
- 1 can rinsed garbanzo beans
- 1 cup chopped and steamed broccoli
- 1 cup cherry tomatoes
- 6 finely sliced radishes
- 4 tbsp pumpkin seeds
- 4 tbsp dried goji berries *optional
- ¼ cup chopped green onions
- ¼ cup chopped parsley
- ¼ cup of Simple Dressing (check recipe under Sauces/Dressings)

Combine ingredients in large bowl and mix! Let sit in refrigerator for 20 minutes. Option: sprinkle pink salt, pepper, kelp seasonings, cayenne pepper, nutritional yeast, and squeeze of lime. Garnish with cubed avocado.

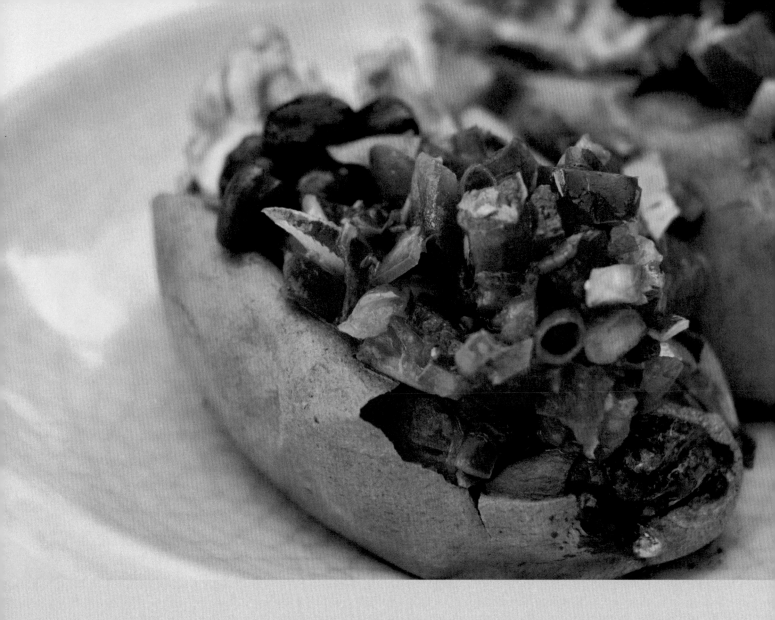

Stuffed Sweet Potato

- 4 large sweet potatoes
- ½ cup chopped chives
- ½ cup black beans
- ¼ cup guacamole
- 1 tbsp nutritional yeast
- ½ cup Homemade Salsa
- Coconut oil, salt and pepper to taste

Preheat oven to 400. Pierce sweet potatoes with fork and place on baking sheet, lined with parchment paper. Bake for 50 minutes. Once out of the oven, slice while hot, put a dab of coconut oil, nutritional yeast, salt and pepper on flesh of potato. Let cool 10 minutes and stuff potatoes with beans, salsa, guacamole, and sprinkle chives.

Meatless "Meatballers"

- ½ cup lentils
- 1-¼ cup veggie broth or water
- ¼ cup chopped scallions
- ½ tsp minced garlic
- ½ cup shredded carrots
- ½ cup soaked and drained walnuts
- ¼ cup almond meal
- 2 tbsp ground flax seeds
- 2 tbsp nutritional yeast
- ½ tsp cumin
- ½ tsp pink salt
- ¼ tsp black pepper
- ½ tsp coconut oil

In a medium pot, heat veggie broth until boiling and add lentils. Then reduce heat and cover for 10-15 minutes until cooked all the way through. Add a little more liquid if they aren't cooked. Once they are, drain any excess off. In a skillet, heat coconut oil (or veggie broth) and add scallions until translucent, add carrots and garlic for another few minutes. Then take all ingredients (including lentils, onions, nuts, herbs) and gradually pour into food processor. Pulse a few times (no need to leave on, a few pulses will do the trick). Mix and mush the ingredients by hand with a wooden spoon. Take mixture and roll into balls the size of a golf ball. Place balls on a baking tray with parchment paper, lightly brush with olive oil if desired. Bake in oven on 350 for 25-30 minutes. Enjoy in a salad, with hummus or with other homemade sauce!

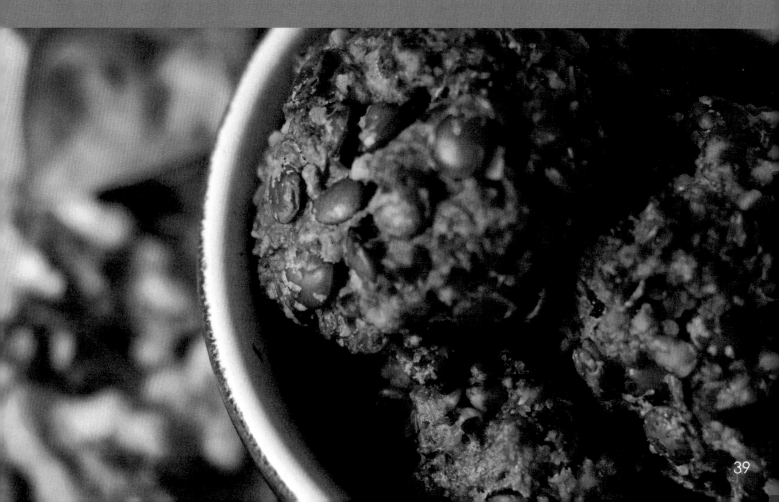

Spring Rolls

- 2-4 rice paper wraps
- 1 medium cucumber
- 1 red pepper
- ¼ finely chopped purple cabbage
- ½ package sprouts *optional
- 1 package tofu
- ½ bunch cilantro
- 4 sprigs basil leaves
- ½ bunch mint
- 1 sliced avocado
- 2 tsp kelp seasonings

Part 1: For the rolls, prep veggies. Chop red pepper and cucumber into 3 inch long, skinny pieces. Place in medium size bowl, and add all other ingredients. For tofu, cut in long and narrow steaks (rectangular). Heat pan with 1 teaspoon coconut oil and a dash of water. Saute tofu to a light golden brown or bake in the oven. Remove from heat and sprinkle kelp seasonings on top. Get rice paper sheets ready (Directions: put warm water in a bowl/plate and place 1 sheet in at a time. Remove and place on cutting board.) Place desired ingredients on top of sheet and roll.

Tip: add avocado slices on top of ingredients before rolling. Keep in mind that it may take some practice to get it right.

*   *   *

Part 2: Dipping Sauce. Mix the following ingredients together in blender. Start with liquids first and then add almond butter and jalapeno. Add salt/pepper to taste.

- ¼ cup almond butter
- 4 tsp tamari
- 3 tbsp lemon juice
- 1 tbsp minced jalapenos
- 1 tsp red chilli flakes
- 1 tsp of honey
- 1 shot of warm water
- 1 tsp of tahini *optional
- 1 tbsp of sesame oil

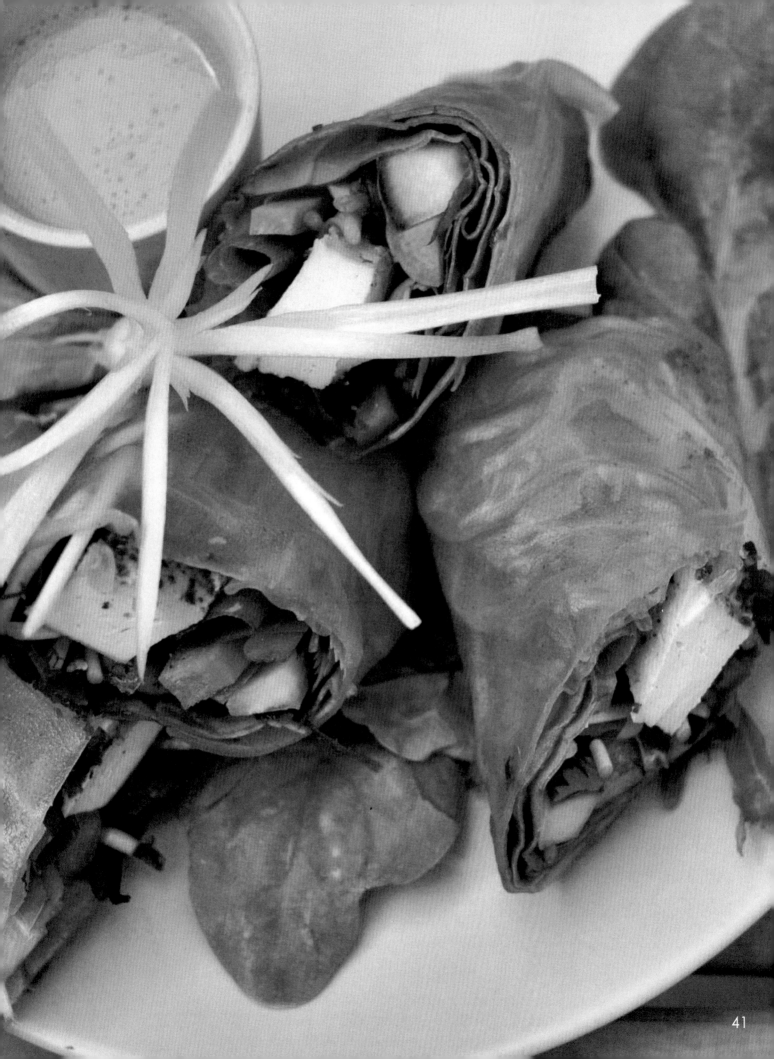

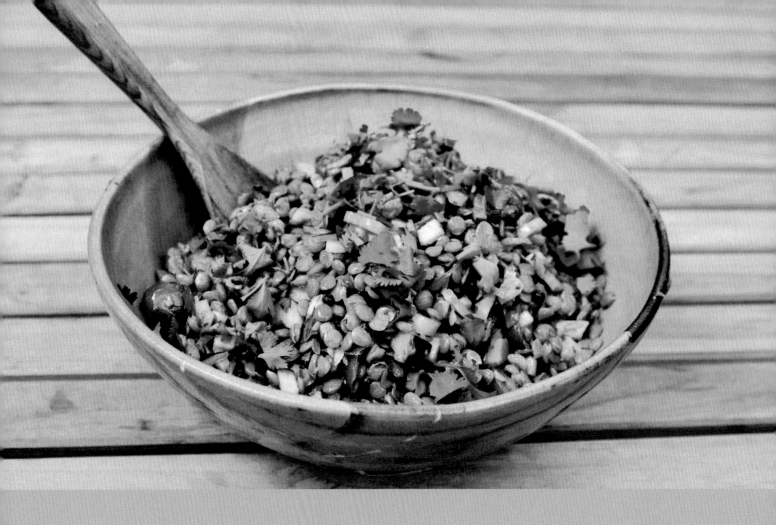

Lentil Salad

- 2 cups cooked lentils
- 1 diced jalapeno
- 1 medium tomato
- ½ cucumber
- ½ red pepper
- ¼ cup cilantro
- ¼ cup green onions
- 2 tbsp coconut amino acids
- 2 tbsp apple-cider vinegar
- 2 tbsp nutritional yeast
- 1 tbsp extra virgin olive oil
- 1 tbsp capers
- seasoning to taste

Chop and dice vegetables together, mix with lentils. Add seasonings like salt, pepper, cayenne, etc. This is a great side or put on top of greens and a scoop of favorite sauce or dressing. I recommend tahini-lemon, Bitchen Sauce, or pesto. Sliced avocado is recommended on most dishes, especially this one!

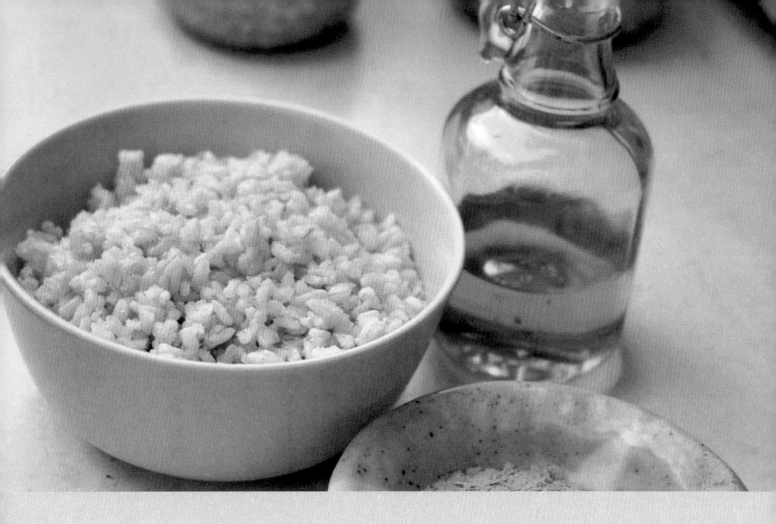

Matty's Rice

- 2 cups water or vegetable broth
- 1 cup arborio rice
- 2 tbsp extra virgin olive oil
- 2 tbsp nutritional yeast
- 1 tbsp Braggs or coconut aminos
- 1 tsp of salt

Bring water to a boil, add rice and reduce heat to low and simmer for 15-20 minutes. Rice should be creamy, with no standing water remaining. Stir in extra virgin olive oil, amino acids, salt and nutritional yeast (for cheesy flavor). Let sit for 10 minutes.

Soups

Coconut Curry Soup

- 1 can coconut milk
- 2 cups veggie stock
- 1 small diced onion
- ½ cups diced carrots
- ¼ cups chopped celery
- ¼ cup diced tomatoes
- ½ cup broccoli
- ⅓ cup snow peas
- 1 chopped zucchini
- 1 tbsp minced garlic
- 1 tbsp minced ginger (or ground)
- 1 tbsp curry powder
- 1 tbsp turmeric
- 1 dried red chili or jalapeno, diced *optional
- 1 stalk of lemongrass *optional
- 2 tbsp coconut oil
- 2-4 bay leaves
- 3 tbsp lime juice

Chop vegetables. Heat coconut oil in large pot over medium fire. Add onions, garlic, ginger, jalapeno, celery, carrots and ½ cup of water. Saute for 5-10 minutes. Add all other veggies, stir for another 10 minutes and add seasonings, bay leaves and then pour in veggie broth. Bring to a boil, add coconut milk and then reduce heat to medium-low. Cover and simmer until all veggies are tender (about 30 minutes), or until ready. Serve warm, stir in lemon juice.

Option: *add 1 cup of brown rice. Add garnish.*
Option: *Garnish with cilantro, mint, basil, mung bean sprouts, dash of cayenne and cumin.*

Veggie Soup

- 1 chopped onion
- ½ inch piece of ginger, minced
- 2 cups celery
- 2 cups carrots
- 1 cup red peppers
- 2 cups butternut squash
- 2 cups sweet potato
- 1 cup zucchini
- 1 cup fresh/frozen peas
- 1 cup fresh/frozen corn
- 4 cups veggie broth
- 1 can diced tomatoes
- 4 bay leaves
- 1 tbsp minced garlic
- ½ tsp pepper
- ½ tsp salt
- 1 tbsp coconut oil
- 1-2 minced jalapenos *optional
- ½ tsp cumin
- ½ tsp paprika
- ½ tsp cayenne
- **Option:** Garnish with finely chopped kale, cilantro, and parsley.

Chop vegetables. Heat coconut oil in large pot over medium heat. Saute onions, garlic, ginger, jalapeno, celery, and carrots for 5-10 minutes. Add all other veggies (except for corn/peas/tomatoes), stir for another 10 minutes and add seasonings, bay leaves, then add tomatoes, vegetable broth and 1 cup of water. Bring to a boil and reduce heat to medium-low. Then, cover and simmer until all veggies are tender about 40 minutes.

Once the soup is ready, throw in peas/corn. Add chopped kale, cilantro, and parsley, when ready to serve. Another great alternative is to add up to 1 cup of cooked quinoa.

Option: Add all ingredients and cook on low for 4 hours in crockpot.

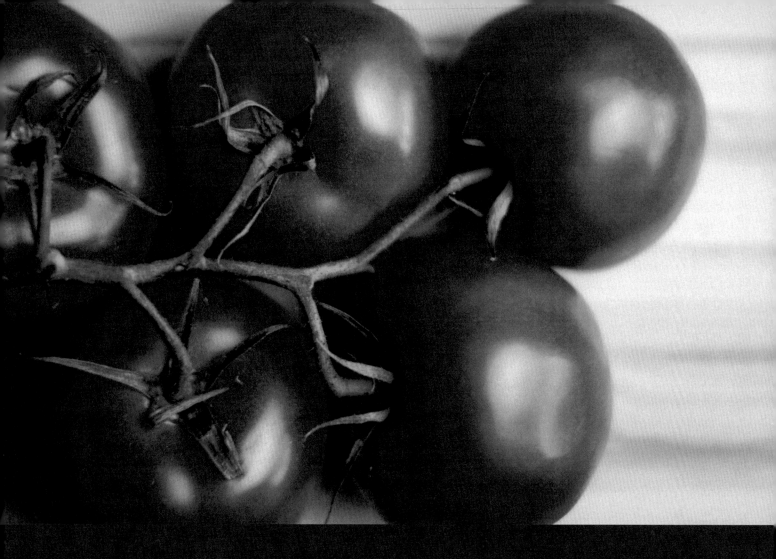

Michelle's Raw Tomato Soup

- 4 cups raw tomatoes
- 2 cups filtered water
- 1 cup soaked and drained cashews
- ½ cup fresh basil
- 4 tbsp extra virgin olive oil
- 2 tbsp nutritional yeast
- 1 tbsp miso paste
- 2 tsp fresh garlic

Combine all ingredients in a high-speed blender or food processor and mix on high until smooth. To warm, blend in a high-speed blender for several more minutes or lightly heat in an uncovered pot on a stove over low heat, being careful not to bring it to a boil.

Easy Lentil Curry

- 1 can rinsed and drained chickpeas
- 1 can coconut milk
- 2 cups frozen peas
- 2 cups lentils
- 1 cup chopped onions
- 1 cup chopped carrots
- 1 ¼ cup vegetable stock
- 2 tbsp coconut oil
- 2 tsp minced garlic
- 1 tbsp sea salt
- 1 tsp cayenne pepper
- 1 tsp cumin
- 1 tsp turmeric
- 1 tbsp curry seasoning
- ¼ cup cilantro or green onions

Place medium saucepan on stove and heat coconut oil (medium/low) and saute onions, garlic, and carrots. Then, add spices once the onions are translucent, turn off momentarily. In separate medium pot, boil vegetable broth, add lentils, and coconut milk. Simmer for 15 minutes on low with lid on, stir as needed, and add water if necessary. Once lentils are cooked, leave heat on low, stir in onion mixture, frozen peas, and can of chickpeas.

Options: *add fresh herbs, chopped spinach, or rice.*

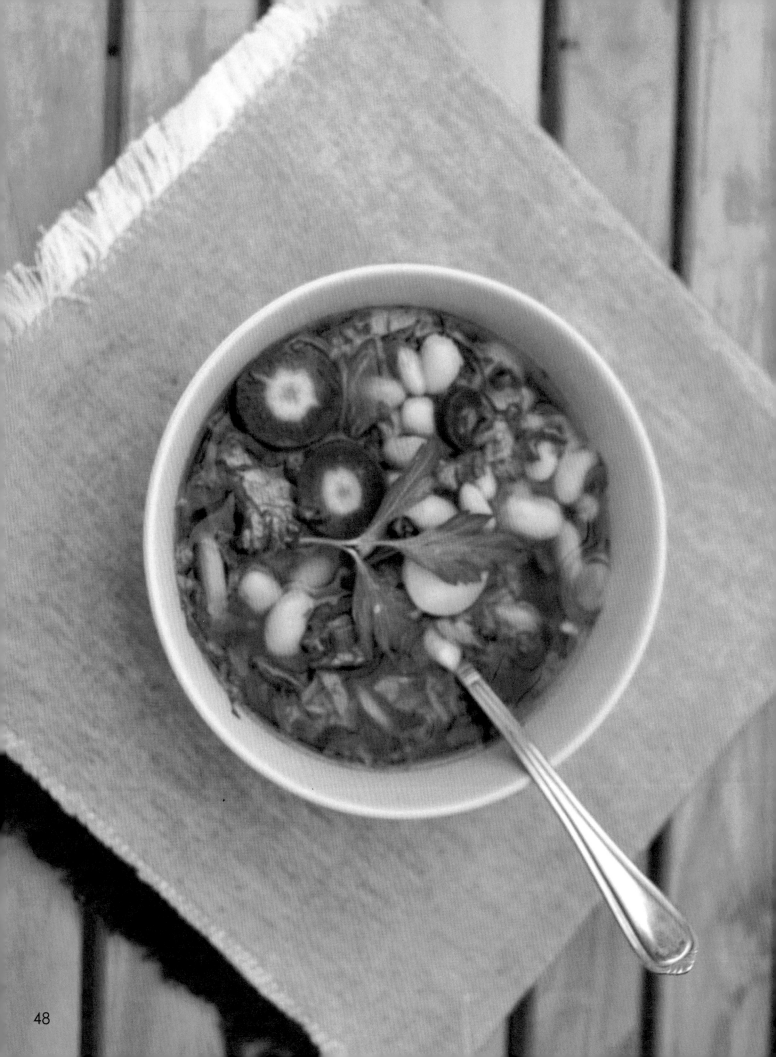

Green & White Soup

- 4-6 cups vegetable broth
- 2 cups finely chopped kale
- 1 can rinsed and drained white beans
- 1 medium diced tomato
- ½ cup chopped carrots
- ½ cup chopped onions
- 1 minced jalapeno
- 2 tsp minced garlic
- 1 tbsp sea salt
- 1 tsp cayenne pepper
- ⅛ tsp rosemary
- ⅛ tsp oregano
- ⅛ tsp thyme
- avocado oil
- nutritional yeast to taste

Place medium saucepan on stove and heat coconut oil (medium/low) and saute onions, garlic, jalapeno and carrot. Then, add spices once the onions are translucent. Stir in tomatoes and beans, stir for a few minutes, and then add vegetable broth. Let simmer for 10 minutes. Turn off heat and add kale. Cover pan with lid and let sit for 5 minutes, before serving. Drizzle avocado oil, pinch of salt, and nutritional yeast on top of individual portions.
Fresh basil is also a delicious garnish.

Salads

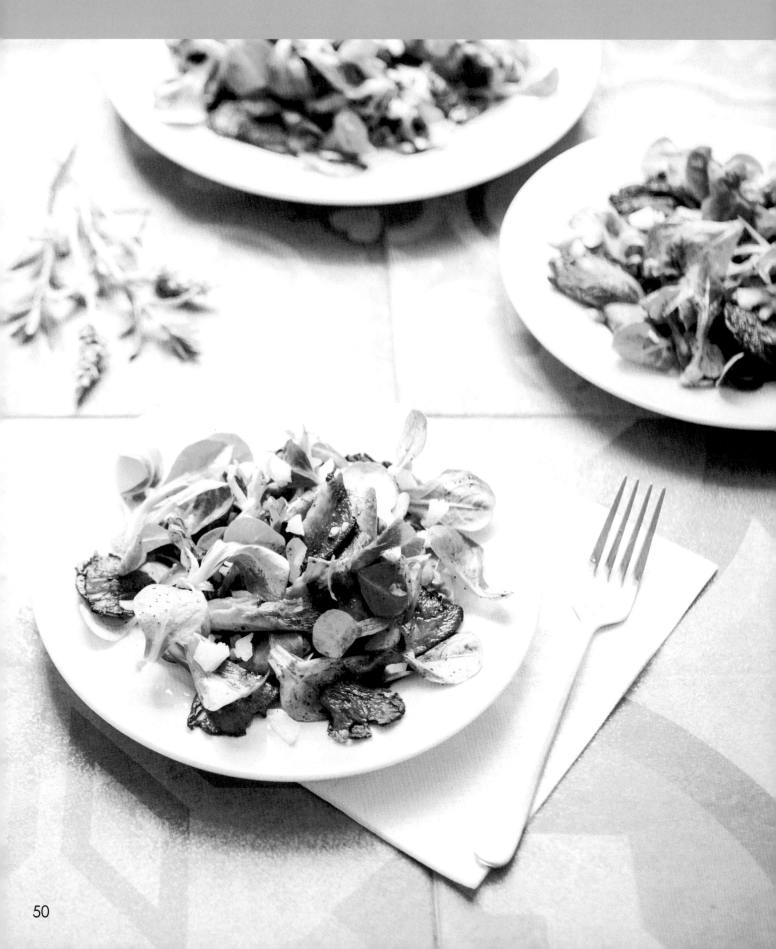

It's a great idea to keep salad ingredients in the fridge at all times. This includes fresh produce like greens, cucumbers, avocados, tomatoes, sprouts, cilantro and other items like cooked quinoa, beans, seeds, nuts, nutritional yeast, etc. Besides homemade salsa, hummus, and salad dressing, I enjoy brightening up my salads with the following...

Pickled Cabbage

- 1 cup finely chopped cabbage
- ½ cup vinegar (white or apple cider)
- ½ cup water
- 1 tsp sea salt
- 1 tsp cayenne
- 1 tsp ginger
- 1 finely chopped jalapeno or clove of garlic

In a medium sized jar, place all ingredients in jar. Shake and let soak in fridge (with lid on tight). Enjoy a few hours later, good 4-5 days.

Carolina's Peruvian Onions

- 5 medium red onions
- 1-2 jalapeno or spicy pepper
- 3 limes
- 2 tbsp olive oil
- 1 tbsp sea salt
- ¼ tsp cayenne
- ¼ tsp cumin

Thinly slice onions and sprinkle salt all over to make them sweat! Let sit for 15 minutes, during that time slice peppers, juice limes and put ingredients in a big glass mason jar. Muddle with other spices if desired and add olive oil. Other fresh herbs like cilantro are also encouraged! Then rinse onions and pat dry with paper towel, add to jar. Muddle and stir all ingredients in the jar and let soak for a few hours, covered and in the refrigerator. Enjoy up to 10 days.

Kale Meets Garbanzo Recipe

- 1 head of kale
- ½ cup cilantro
- 10 cherry tomatoes
- 1 can rinsed garbanzo beans
- 4 tbsp lemon juice
- 4 tbsp pumpkin seeds
- ½ sliced avocado
- extra virgin olive oil
- ¼ tsp cayenne
- ¼ tsp cumin
- ¼ tsp paprika
- pink salt and pepper to taste

Pre-heat oven to 400. Wash kale, dry and chop. Place in medium sized bowl and massage with squeezed lemon and 1 tbsp extra virgin olive oil for a few minutes. Drain and rinse garbanzo beans, place in small bowl. Mix 1 tbsp of oil and spices until beans are covered.
Place beans on a pan with foil or wax paper. Put in the oven for 20 minutes. Take out and let cool. Add tomatoes, cilantro, beans, avocado, and seeds to kale.

Kale Salad Recipe

- 6 cup roughly chopped kale
- 1 package of cherry tomatoes
- ¼ cup lemon juice
- 1-2 tbsp extra virgin olive oil

In a medium sized bowl, massage 2 bunches of chopped kale with 1 tablespoon of oil and lemon juice.

Dressing: *In a blender or food processor, add the following ingredients.*
Tip: Start with liquids at the bottom first, gradually add almond butter, onion, garlic, cilantro, avocado, etc.

- 2 tbsp filtered water
- 1 tbsp unfiltered apple cider vinegar
- 1 tbsp extra virgin olive oil
- 1 tbsp honey
- 1-2 tbsp of coconut amino acids
- ½ lemon
- ¾ jar of almond butter
- 1 bunch of cilantro stems (throw leaves in with kale)
- 2 cloves garlic
- ⅓ finely chopped onion
- 1 jalapeno
- 1 avocado
Notes: Add a splash of water if you need.

Add dressing to kale with salt/pepper to taste. Add ½ chopped avocado and baby tomatoes and mix together. This salad will keep for a few days. Serves 4-6.

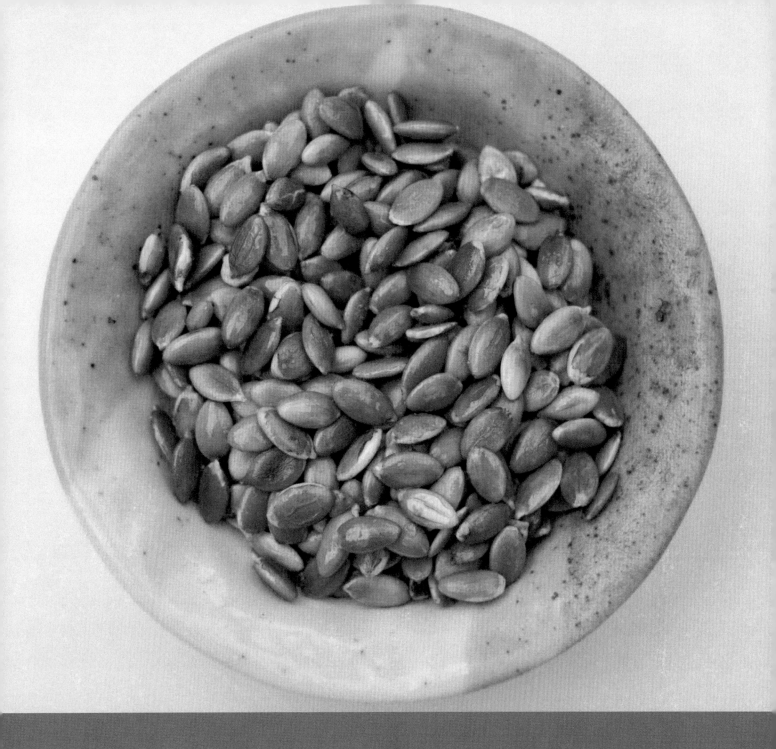

Powerful Pumpkin Seeds

- 1 cup raw pumpkin seeds
- ½ tbsp coconut oil
- Pinch of sea salt

Heat coconut oil in small sauce pan until melted. Add pumpkin seeds and stir until they turn a light golden brown, add salt or any other spices desired.

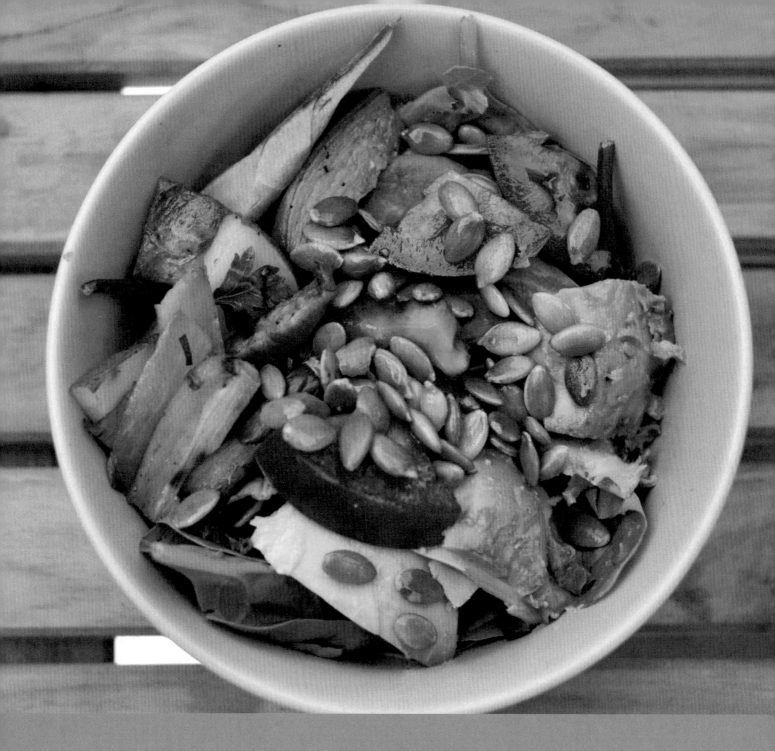

Mixed Greens Salad

Place ingredients in a bowl, mix and serve. Use dressing of choice.

- 4 cups of spring mix
- 3 cups of roasted veggies
- ¼ avocado
- ½ medium tomato diced
- 1-2 tbsp of seeds or chopped nuts
- Choice of protein and dressing

Baked Tofu Salad

- 6 cup spring mix
- 1 cup cooked quinoa
- ¼ cup chopped parsley
- ¼ cup chopped green onion
- ½ green
- ½ yellow bell pepper
- 1 package of firm tofu
- 1 pound cherry tomatoes
- 1 roughly chopped, baked sweet potato

Optional add-ons: pumpkin seeds, hemp hearts, avocado, sprouts, nutritional yeast, etc.

Baked Tofu: Slice tofu into 3 layers and cut into 1 ½ inch squares. Marinate tofu for minimum 30 minutes (or more), each side, in 1 tablespoon olive oil, 2 tablespoons of tamari and a few shakes of the following seasonings: curry powder, cayenne, paprika, cumin, onion, garlic, turmeric, pink salt, pepper. Place in glass cookware in oven on 375, let bake 15-20 minutes, flip each piece and cook for an additional 15 minutes. Remove and let cool.

In the meantime, place tomatoes, bell peppers, quinoa, parsley, green onion, baked sweet potato, on top of greens. Place tofu and additional toppings over salad.

Tunafish, Tunafish, MOCK Tunafish

This recipe is great for salad topping, dip, or in a wrap (coconut wrap, nori, or chard).
Tip: Soak seeds for 2 hours and strain.

- 1 cup soaked, raw sunflower seeds
- ¼ cup lemon juice
- 1-3 tbsp mustard with seeds
- 1 tbsp raw apple cider vinegar
- 1 tbsp coconut amino acids
- 1-2 tsp minced garlic

Place ingredients listed above in a blender, add water if needed. Sprinkle salt, pepper, cayenne, cumin to taste. Remove and place in medium sized bowl, then add the following:

- ½ finely chopped cucumber
- 4 stalks finely chopped celery
- ¼ cup finely chopped dill
- 5 sprigs of cilantro
- 2-3 tbsp capers
- 1-2 tbsp kelp seasonings
- 2 tbsp raw pumpkin seeds
Option to add 1 finely chopped green apple

Apple Choy Slaw

- 6 cups chopped bok choy
- ½ cup alfalfa sprouts
- ¼ cup thinly sliced small red onion
- ¼ cup sliced green apple
- 1 avocado

Dressing
- ¼ cup extra virgin olive oil
- 3 tbsp raw apple cider vinegar
- 3 tbsp coconut amino acids
- 2 tsp honey
- 1 tsp ground coriander
- 1 tsp dijon mustard
- salt and pepper to taste

Combine all ingredients in a bowl. Prepare dressing in a bowl or jar and mix well. Pour dressing over salad. Eat immediately. If serving the salad later, add the apples and avocado just before, to prevent them from browning.

Options: *Try cabbage instead of bok choy or carrot slices instead of onion. Add fresh herbs such as cilantro, parsley, mint or scallions. Double the dressing ingredients and use on leftover grains.*

Cool As A Cucumber Salad

- 3 large cucumbers
- 2 carrot
- 1 red bell pepper
- ½ white onion
- ½ avocado
- 3-4 tbsp raw apple cider vinegar
- 2 tbsp tamari
- 2 tbsp sesame seeds
- Pink salt and pepper to taste

Chop cucumbers and peppers and place in a bowl. Grate carrots and finely chop onion and add to the mix. Toss and sprinkle with sea salt, let sit for 10 minutes. Sprinkle with vinegar and tamari, then chill for 2 to 4 hours, serve with avocado and sesame seeds when ready to eat.

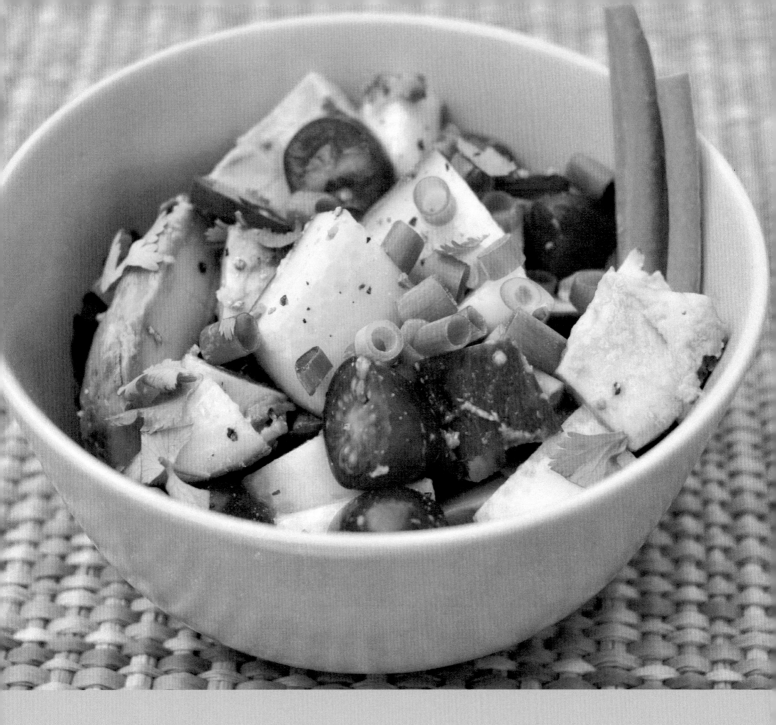

Cucumber, Tomato, Avo Salad

Mix the following ingredients in small bowl, and enjoy as a meal or side salad. And add pink salt, pepper and cayenne to taste.

- 1 medium cubed cucumber
- 2 cubed tomatoes
- 1 cubed avocado
- ¼ cup green onion
- 2 tbsp lemon juice
- 1 tbsp extra virgin olive oil
- 1 tbsp coconut amino acids

Autumn Arugula Salad

- 6 cups baby arugula
- 1 cup pomegranate seeds
- 1 cup sliced, seedless cucumber
- 1 acorn squash
- 1 sliced avocado
- ¼ cup chopped pecans
- 2 tbsp coconut oil
- 1 tbsp pumpkin seeds
- 1 tsp of honey
- ¼ tsp pink salt
- ¼ tsp pumpkin pie spice

Cut acorn squash in half, remove seeds, and then slice into ½ inch pieces (in the shape of a letter C). In a large skillet over medium heat, add coconut oil. Once it melts add squash slices with salt and pepper. Place in skillet and cook until golden; about 5 minutes per side. In a small saucepan over low heat, add ½ tsp of coconut oil, let melt and then add pecans. Shake the pan for about 5 minutes until golden and sprinkle pumpkin pie spice seasoning. Modify to your liking (cinnamon, clove, ginger, etc).

In a large bowl, place arugula, avocado, pomegranate seeds, cucumber, pecans and squash pieces. Sprinkle with salt, pepper, and pomegranate ginger vinaigrette.

*Pomegranate Ginger Vinaigrette recipe can be found in the Dressings & Sauces section.

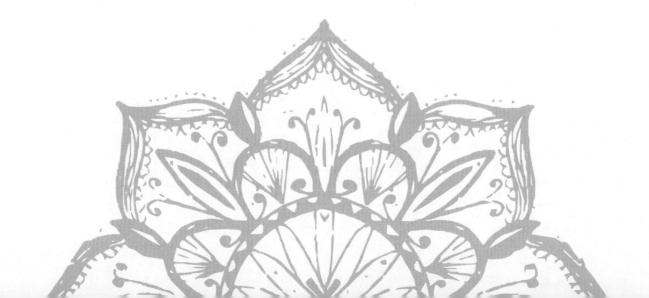

Dressings & Sauces

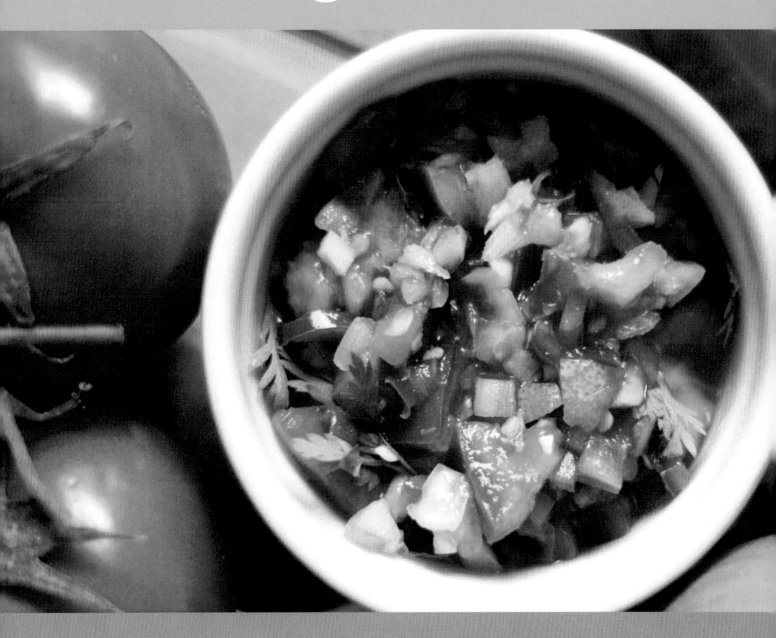

The following recipes use a blender or food processor if desired! Option to blend ingredients together until creamy. Otherwise, for dressings that aren't blended, place all ingredients in jar, except olive oil. Take one tablespoon of dressing and add one tablespoon of olive oil the day you use it. That way, the olive oil doesn't harden in the fridge. If dressings or sauces are too thick, add a little filtered water.

Simple Dressing

- 1 cup lemon juice
- ⅓ cup extra virgin olive oil
- 6 tbsp coconut amino acids
- 2 tbsp raw apple cider vinegar
- ¼ cup finely chopped onion
- 2 tbsp minced garlic
- 1 tbsp mustard
- 1 tbsp honey
- 1 tbsp chia seeds

A few sprinkles of salt, pepper, cayenne, rosemary, parsley, cilantro.
Put ingredients in small mason jar, stir and shake as needed.

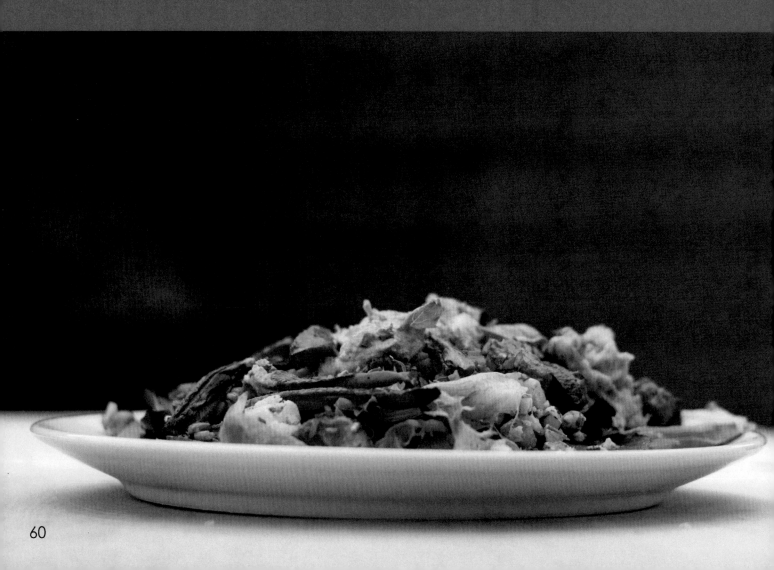

Lemon Poppyseed Dressing

Put ingredients in small mason jar, stir and shake as needed.

- ½ cup extra virgin olive oil
- 3 tbsp lemon juice
- 1 tbsp poppy seeds
- 1 tbsp maple
- 1 tbsp dijon mustard

Asian Dressing

Put ingredients in small mason jar, stir and shake as needed.

- ⅓ cup extra virgin olive oil
- ⅓ cup flax seed oil
- ¼ cup rice vinegar
- ¼ cup water
- 3 tbsp raw apple cider vinegar
- 3 tbsp honey
- 2 tbsp minced garlic
- 2 tsp minced ginger
- 1 tbsp sesame seeds

Tahini Lemon Dressing

Mix in blender. First place liquid ingredients in and slowly add yeast and garlic in until creamy.

- ¼ cup tahini
- ½ cup fresh lemon juice
- ¼ cup nutritional yeast
- 3 tbsp extra virgin olive oil
- 1 clove garlic

Carrot Ginger Dressing

Put ingredients in small mason jar, stir and shake as needed.

- 1 cup grated carrot
- ¼ cup extra virgin olive oil
- 3 tbsp apple cider vinegar
- 2 tbsp maple
- 1 tbsp peeled & minced ginger
- 1 tbsp tamari
- 1 tbsp miso paste
- 1 tsp sesame oil
- 2-4 tsp water

Grapefruit Vinaigrette

Put ingredients in small mason jar, stir and shake as needed.

- ½ cup grapefruit juice
- ¼ cup avocado oil
- 1 tbsp mustard powder
- 1 tbsp maple syrup
- ¼ tsp sea salt
- 1 tbsp chia seeds

Pomegranate Ginger Vinaigrette

Combine above ingredients into small mason jar and shake with lid on. Store in the fridge for up to one week.

- ⅓ cup extra virgin olive oil
- ⅓ cup pomegranate juice
- ¼ cup raw apple cider vinegar
- ½ tsp freshly grated ginger
- 1 tsp minced garlic
- ¼ tsp pink salt
- ¼ tsp pepper

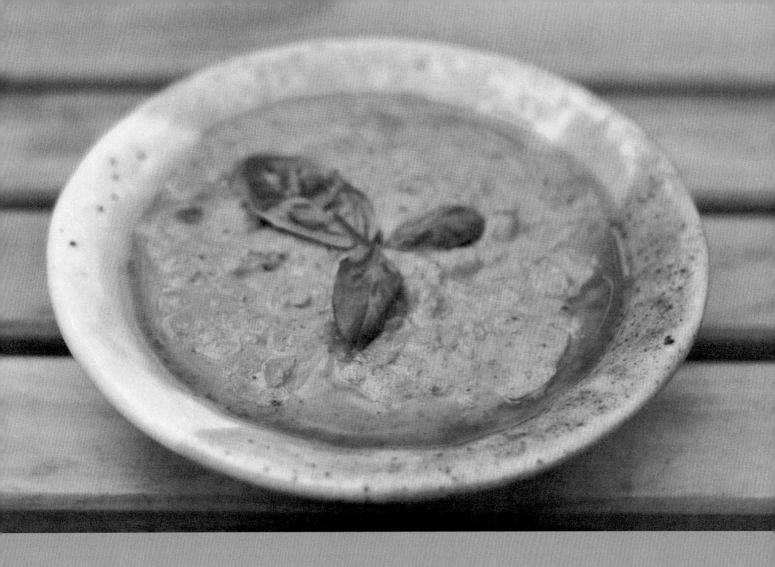

Basil Dressing

- ¼ cup extra virgin olive oil
- ½ cup soaked walnuts
- 1 handful of basil
- 3-4 tbsp water
- 3 tsp lemon juice
- 1 tbsp minced garlic
- 1 tbsp maple
- ¼ tsp sea salt

A few sprinkles of salt, pepper, cayenne, rosemary, parsley, cilantro.
Put ingredients in small mason jar, stir and shake as needed.

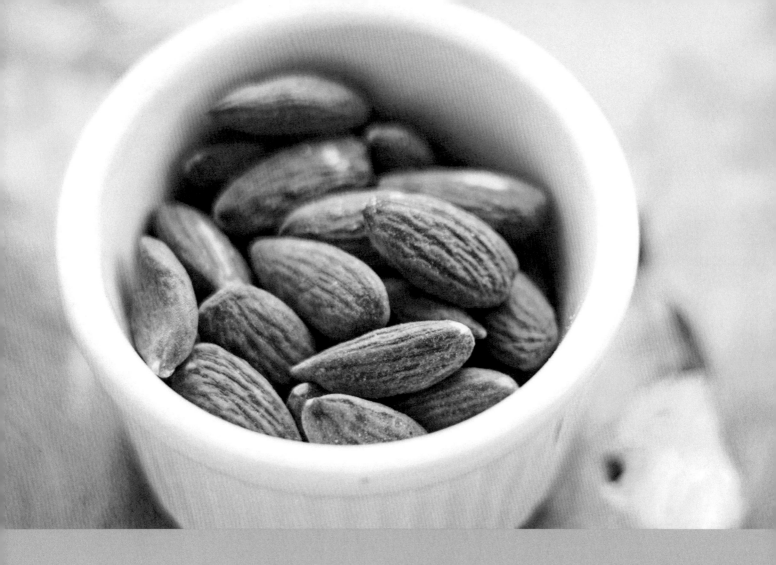

Bitchen Sauce

- ¾ cup raw almonds (soaked overnight)
- ¾ cup filtered water
- ¼ cup olive oil
- ¼ cup grapeseed oil
- ¼ cup lemon juice (about 1 ½ lemons)
- 3 tbsp nutritional yeast
- 2 tbsp minced garlic
- 2 tsp bragg liquid aminos
- ½ tsp salt
- ½ tsp cumin
- 1 tsp chili powder
- ¼ tsp coriander
- ¼ tsp paprika
- 1 handful fresh organic cilantro.

Place all ingredients in high speed blender. Slowly blend for one minute. Turn the dial up to high, and continue to blend for 1-2 minutes or until smooth and creamy. Store in the refrigerator or freezer. Sauce may separate so just stir up when serving.

Pesto Recipe

Throw ingredients into blender/ food processor. Put the liquids in first and gradually add other ingredients. Add a shot of water if it needs more liquid. Pesto is an easy sauce to have around for GF pasta, roasted/raw vegetables, etc.

- 1 cup fresh basil
- ½ cup spinach
- ¾ cup pine nuts (or soaked almonds/walnuts)
- ¼ cup nutritional yeast
- ¼ cup extra virgin olive oil
- ¼ cup lemon juice
- 3 tbsp minced garlic
- pink salt and pepper to taste

Carrot Top Pesto

Pulse ingredients in blender or food processor.

- 1 cup fresh basil
- 1 bundle of carrot tops
- ¾ cup pine nuts (or soaked walnuts)
- ¼ cup nutritional yeast
- ¼ cup extra virgin olive oil
- ¼ cup lemon juice
- 3 tbsp minced garlic
- pink salt and pepper to taste

Option: add ½ avocado for extra creaminess.

Avocado salsa

Mix the following ingredients, add to salad or use as a snack with raw vegetables.

- 2 cubed avocados
- 1 diced tomato
- 1 can rinsed and drained black beans
- 1 finely chopped jalapeno
- 4 tbsp lime juice
- 2 tbsp extra virgin olive oil
- 2 tbsp raw apple cider vinegar
- 1 tbsp coconut amino acids
- 1 finely chopped red onion
- ¼ cup chopped cilantro
- 1 tsp red pepper flakes
- 1 tsp cumin
- ½ tsp pink salt
- ½ tsp pepper

Cauliflower Mash

- 1 head of cauliflower
- 1 cup of vegetable broth
- ½ cup coconut milk
- ½ cup soaked raw cashews
- 4 tbsp nutritional yeast
- 3 tbsp extra virgin olive oil
- 2 tbsp coconut amino acids
- 2 tbsp lemon juice
- 1 tbsp minced garlic

Warm up vegetable broth in pot on medium-high. Chop cauliflower and place in pot with lid to steam for 5-7 minutes, or until tender. In a blender, place all other ingredients in (cashews drained), blend and add cauliflower with broth in it. Add salt and pepper to taste. If it needs more liquid to blend, add more coconut milk or veggie broth.
This cauliflower mash can be transformed into a fabulous sauce for gluten-free pasta, vegetable dip, or dressing. Add coconut milk to make creamier. Option to leave 1 cup in the blender and add a handful of cilantro, a dash of lemon juice and one avocado. Blend together to make a creamy green sauce. This sauce can be served hot or cold.

Ashley's Special Sauce

- 2 cups cherry tomatoes
- ¼ cup chopped red bell pepper
- ¼ cup soaked raw cashews
- 3 dehydrated sun dried tomatoes
- 2 tbsp extra virgin olive oil
- 1 tbsp coconut oil
- 1 small carrot
- Sea salt to taste

Blacken the tomatoes over high heat in large sauce pan on the stove for 7 minute (or until blackened). Add red pepper to the same pan using no oil, for 5 more minutes. Transfer tomatoes and bell pepper to a high powered blender and add all the remaining ingredients except the sea salt. The sun dried tomatoes will add a fair amount of salt so blend first and then add accordingly.

Hummus
- 1 can drained and rinsed chickpeas
- ¼ cup filtered water
- ¼ cup lemon juice
- 2 tbsp extra virgin olive oil
- 1 tbsp minced garlic
- ½ tsp cumin
- **Option** to add tahini

Garnish with roasted pine nuts and paprika. For additional kick, I throw in chopped ginger. Put ingredients in a food processor/high powered blender. If needed, add water. Pink salt and pepper to taste.

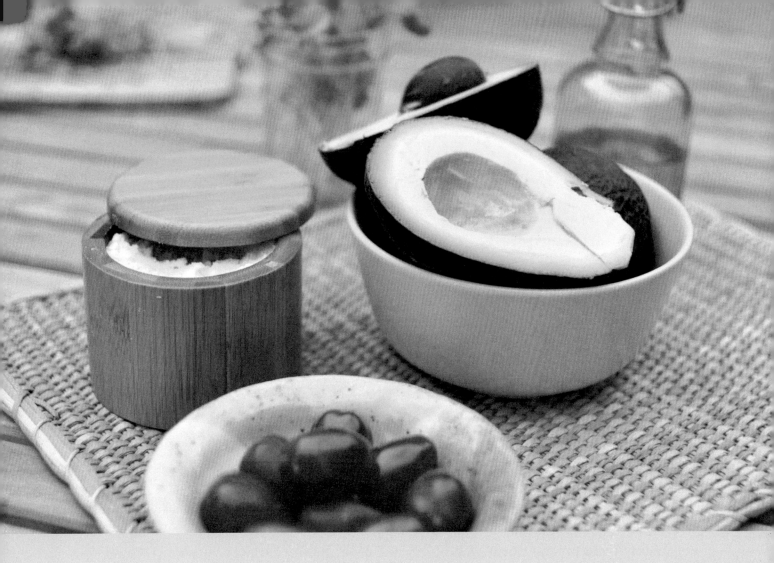

Yummy Guacamole

Mix the following ingredients until creamy and add to salad or use as a snack with raw veggies.

- 3 cubed avocados
- ¼ cup diced tomato
- ¼ cup chopped cilantro
- ¼ cup finely chopped onion
- ¾ cup finely chopped celery
- 2 tbsp lime juice
- 2 tsp minced garlic
- 1 finely chopped jalapeno
- 1 tsp cumin
- ½ tsp pink salt
- ½ tsp pepper

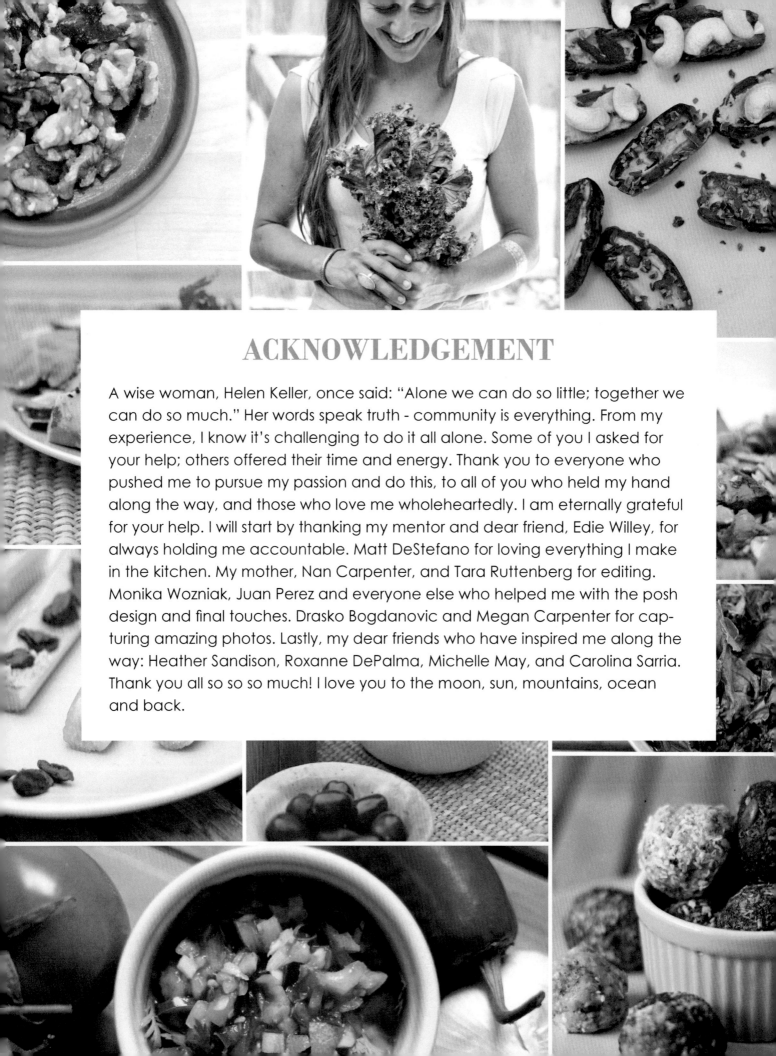

ACKNOWLEDGEMENT

A wise woman, Helen Keller, once said: "Alone we can do so little; together we can do so much." Her words speak truth - community is everything. From my experience, I know it's challenging to do it all alone. Some of you I asked for your help; others offered their time and energy. Thank you to everyone who pushed me to pursue my passion and do this, to all of you who held my hand along the way, and those who love me wholeheartedly. I am eternally grateful for your help. I will start by thanking my mentor and dear friend, Edie Willey, for always holding me accountable. Matt DeStefano for loving everything I make in the kitchen. My mother, Nan Carpenter, and Tara Ruttenberg for editing. Monika Wozniak, Juan Perez and everyone else who helped me with the posh design and final touches. Drasko Bogdanovic and Megan Carpenter for capturing amazing photos. Lastly, my dear friends who have inspired me along the way: Heather Sandison, Roxanne DePalma, Michelle May, and Carolina Sarria. Thank you all so so so much! I love you to the moon, sun, mountains, ocean and back.

Made in the USA
San Bernardino, CA
11 January 2017